CLINICAL REASONING

THE ART AND SCIENCE OF CRITICAL AND CREATIVE THINKING

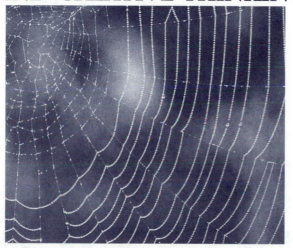

Annike —
Best to you
as you venture into the
reason into the
future —
Donald Rosseto

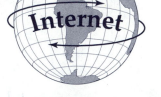

CLINICAL REASONING

THE ART AND SCIENCE OF CRITICAL AND CREATIVE THINKING

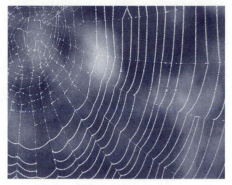

Daniel J. Pesut PhD, RN, CS, FAAN
Professor and Department Chairperson
Environments for Health
Indiana University School of Nursing

JoAnne Herman PhD, RN, CSME
Associate Professor University of South Carolina
College of Nursing

Delmar Publishers

an International Thomson Publishing company I(T)P®

Albany • Bonn • Boston • Cincinnati • Detroit • London • Madrid
Melbourne • Mexico City • New York • Pacific Grove • Paris • San Francisco
Singapore • Tokyo • Toronto • Washington

Cover Design: Scott Keidong

Delmar Staff

Publisher: William Brottmiller
Acquisitions Editor: Cathy L. Esperti
Developmental Editor: Patricia A. Gaworecki
Production Coordinator: James Zayicek
Art and Design Coordinator: Timothy J. Conners

COPYRIGHT © 1999
By Delmar Publishers
a division of International Thomson Publishing Inc.
I︎T︎P︎ The ITP logo is a trademark under license.
Printed in the United States of America

For more information, contact:

Delmar Publishers
3 Columbia Circle, Box 15015
Albany, New York 12212-5015

Nelson Canada
1120 Birchmount Road
Scarborough, Ontario
M1K 5G4 Canada

**International Thompson
Publishing Asia**
60 Albert St.
Albert Complex #15-01
Singapore 189969

**International Thomson Publishing
Europe**
Berkshire House
168-173 High Holborn
London, WC1V 7AA
United Kingdom

**International Thomson
Editores**
Seneca 53
Colonia Polanco
11560 Mexico D. F. Mexico

**International Thompson
Publishing—Japan**
Hirakawacho Kyowa Building, 3F
2-2-1 Hirakawacho Chiyoda-Ku
Tokyo 102 Japan

Nelson ITP Australia
102 Dodds Street
South Melbourne
Victoria, 3205 Australia

**International Thompson
Publishing GmbH**
Konigswinterer Strasse 418
53227 Bonn
Germany

2 3 4 5 6 7 8 9 10   XXX   03 02 01 00 99

Library of Congress Cataloging-in-Publication Data

Pesut, Daniel J.
    Clinical reasoning : the art and science of critical and creative
thinking / Daniel J. Pesut, JoAnne Herman.
        p.   cm.
    Includes bibliographical references and index.
    ISBN 0-8273-7869-6
    1. Nursing diagnosis.   2. Nursing—Decision making.   3. Clinical
medicine—Decision making.   4. Clinical competence.   5. Diagnosis,
Differential.   I. Herman, JoAnne.   II. Title.
    RT48.6.P47 1999
610.73—dc21   98-37445
                                                                  CIP

Contents

Preface

Teaching clinical reasoning over the past 28 years has provided us with the opportunity to analyze and evaluate the nursing process and observe its development over time. We have identified three distinct generations of nursing process (Pesut & Herman, 1998). Each generation was influenced by the state of knowledge development and contemporary forces operative during its formation. The first generation (1950–1970) focused on problems and process. The second generation (1970–1990) highlighted diagnosis and reasoning. The third generation we see emerging underscores the importance of outcome specification and testing.

Based on our work with students in clinical reasoning courses, we have created and developed the outcome-present state-test (OPT) model of clinical reasoning. OPT is a third-generation nursing process model that emphasizes reflection, outcome specification, and testing, given the nature of a client's or patient's story. The model supports the application of critical and creative thinking in clinical practice. In this book we present and explain the OPT model of clinical reasoning.

The OPT model is a concurrent, iterative model of clinical reasoning. Reflection is an essential part of the reasoning process. We have done our best to define the thinking strategies and techniques we believe are the essential ingredients of clinical reasoning and reflection. We outline the role of critical and creative thinking skills that support the reflective reasoning core of the model. The model uses the facts associated with a client's story to frame the context and content for clinical reasoning. Clinical decision making in this model is defined as choosing nursing actions. Clinical judgments are the conclusions drawn from tests that compare client present-state data to specified outcome-state criteria. Concurrent judgments related to the match or mismatch of present-state and outcome-state data result in the need for clinical decisions. Clinical judgments are derived from the meaning one gives to outcome evidence of tests created. Reflections on judgments suggest the need for reframing the situation, creation of new tests, and additional clinical decisions or judgments about other types of tests needed for outcome achievement. Many experienced clinicians tell us the model makes sense.

Use and application of the OPT model helps identify some of the covert thinking skills nurses use to reason about clinical care outcomes. By making the processes and thinking strategies more explicit, one can "unpack" the thinking used in clinical reasoning. Making these strategies more explicit has several benefits. Such analysis is likely to help teachers teach, students learn, and clinicians reason better. The focus on outcomes provides direction for care and benefits clients. A brief overview of the chapters in the book will orient the reader.

In Chapter 1 we discuss the art and science of nursing in the context of social policies. Specifically, we highlight the American Association of Colleges of Nursing vision for nursing education and the Pew Health Profession Commission competencies for future health care practitioners. We emphasize the importance of reflection, responsibility, and knowledge work for the development of clinical reasoning competence. We introduce and reinforce the value of an inquisitive clinical reasoning attitude and client stories as a foundation for clinical reasoning.

In Chapter 2 we define and trace the evolution of three generations of nursing process. We compare and contrast differences among the scientific method, problem solving, traditional nursing process, and the OPT model.

In Chapter 3 we introduce key terms associated with the OPT model and discuss differences between problem-oriented and outcome-oriented thinking as well as contrasts between academic and practical intelligence. The importance of client stories and framing is discussed in the context of critical and creative thinking, reflexive reasoning, and thinking strategies that support reasoning. Knowledge work and the value of a clinical vocabulary for reasoning are highlighted. A case study is used to illustrate key points and application of OPT model differences.

Building on the importance of knowledge work and the need for a clinical vocabulary, Chapter 4 is devoted to a discussion about knowledge work in nursing. Levels of nursing practice data are explained. Work of the North American Nursing Diagnosis Association Classification of Nursing Diagnoses (NANDA), the Iowa Nursing Intervention Classification Project (NIC), Nursing Sensitive Outcomes Classification (NOC), the Omaha classification system, Marjory Gordon's functional health patterns, and the *Diagnostic Statistical Manual of Mental Disorders-IV* are reviewed.

Unit II is series of case studies that illustrate how the OPT model is used to support clinical reasoning across contexts. In Chapter 5 we introduce tools and techniques that support the OPT model. For example, the OPT Model Worksheet and Clinical Reasoning Web help people grasp critical and creative thinking relationships among ideas, concepts, and reasoning strategies. Use of case studies illustrates analysis and application of the following thinking strategies that support clinical reasoning: knowledge work, self-talk, prototype identification, schema search, hypothesizing, if–then thinking, comparative analysis, juxtaposing, reflexive comparison, reframing, and reflection check. A Thinking Strategies Worksheet is provided in each chapter for you to use in learning and tracking your understanding and use of these strategies and techniques.

Chapter 6 presents a case for clinical reasoning with a wellness focus in a primary care context. Chapter 7 focuses on a case study in an acute care context. Chapter 8 illustrates application of the OPT model in a home health situation. Chapter 9 examines a case in a community mental health context. Chapter 10 illustrates the use and application of the OPT model with a person who is in a long-term care context. In each of these examples we follow a similar format: we introduce the client story, discuss the nursing knowledge classification system of choice (given the context), show how to spin and weave a Clinical Reasoning Web, and then discuss the thinking strategies that support reflective clinical reasoning and how clinical decisions, judgments, and reflections about the case evolve. A completed OPT Model Worksheet is included in each chapter. Each case is also accompanied by a Thinking Strategies Worksheet that challenges readers to find and document examples from their own thinking about the case presented.

In Unit III three chapters describe alternative uses and applications of the OPT model. In Chapter 11 a discussion of academic, practical, nursing, and successful intelligence is developed. Use of the OPT model to support clinical supervision is reinforced through the use of 20 questions that guide the supervision process with OPT.

In Chapter 12 a discussion of practice theory and science supports the innovation of using OPT for structuring middle-range theories for nursing practice. Finally, Chapter 13 discusses future trends and health care consequences. Contributions of the OPT model of reflective clinical reasoning to future educational and research and practice agendas for a theory of clinical reasoning are discussed.

The OPT model builds on the traditional nursing process, but is different from the nursing process in several ways. First, the OPT model organizes client needs and nursing care activities around a keystone issue. If keystone issues are resolved, then many of the more peripheral problems will resolve themselves. Second, the OPT model makes explicit the juxtaposition of a present state with a well-defined outcome state. The juxtapositioning or side-by-side consideration of present and outcome states creates differences that we call tests. Test conditions activate clinical decisions and evidence-based judgments. Third, the model reinforces the concurrent, iterative characteristics of clinical reasoning. Fourth, the OPT model is compatible with an outcome-driven health care systems because it is built on a foundation of critical thinking and reflective judgment. The OPT model supports teaching and learning of clinical reasoning, clinical supervision, and middle-range theory development. The structure and application of the model, definition of terms, and thinking strategies that support use of the model have educational, practice, and research consequences for contemporary nursing. Clinicians, educators, managers, and administrators are invited to consider the OPT model as an evolutionary development of traditional nursing process.

Daniel J. Pesut
Carmel, Indiana

JoAnne Herman
Columbia, South Carolina
August 1998

REFERENCE

Pesut, D., & Herman, J. (1998). OPT: Transformation of nursing process for contemporary practice. *Nursing Outlook, 46*(1), 29–36.

Dedication

To those who believe nursing is art and science and know in their hearts that caring involves critical and creative thinking in the context of a patient's story

Acknowledgments

Many people have supported and nurtured the incubation and development of this project. Most importantly, we are grateful for the support and encouragement we have received from our families. Susan Ziel, Elliott, Erin, and Donna Pesut were with us in so many ways. Wayne and Jennifer Herman were faithful cheerleaders. We are grateful to Dr. Bob Jannarone, who planted the seed and introduced us to the ideas of concurrent information processing. Robert Dilts and members of the NLP World Health Community stimulated and encouraged the vision and mission associated with the production of this book. Drs. Mary Frame and Phyllis Kritek modeled the leadership and courage to persevere. Finally, many individuals provided content and creative support. Special thanks to all of the students and the registered nurse students in the clinical reasoning courses at the University of South Carolina College of Nursing, Tammy Simpson, Lisa Spruill, June Headley, Mary Alice Stein, and Charles Harris. We also want to thank our guides in the publishing world, Patty Gaworecki and Cathy Esperti. Special kudos to the folks at Delmar Publishers who are dedicated to the art and science of nursing. The following reviewers provided valuable feedback throughout the production of this title:

Connie Short Lowry, MS, RN, CCRN, CNS
Clinical Nurse Specialist
Nursing Faculty
University of Central Oklahoma
Edmond, Oklahoma

Dr. Joanne McCloskey, PhD, RN, FAAN
Distinguished Professor of Nursing
College of Nursing
University of Iowa
Iowa City, Iowa

Rosemary Kellar PhD, MSN, RN
Clinical Instructor
University of South Florida
College of Nursing
Tampa, Florida

Helen Erikson, PhD, RN, HNC, FAAN
Emeritus Professor
The University of Texas at Austin
Austin, Texas

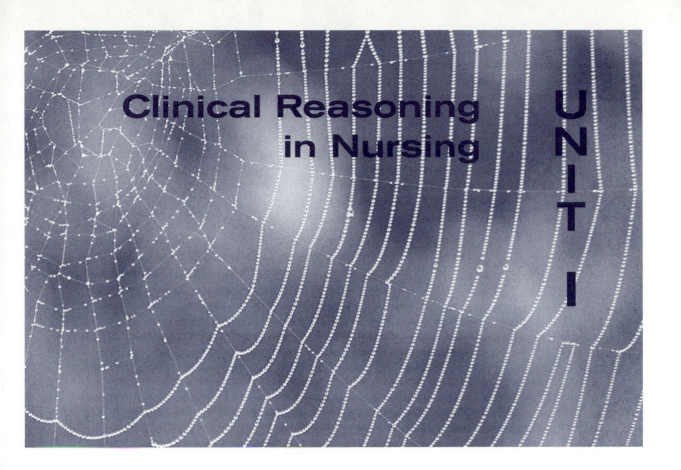

Clinical Reasoning in Nursing

UNIT I

Unit I is comprised of four chapters. In Chapter 1, we discuss the role of nursing in society and the importance of thinking and reasoning in nursing practice. In Chapter 2, we trace the history of the nursing process and discuss how this process has undergone changes and transformations through time. Three generations of nursing process are described. In Chapter 3, we introduce and explain the outcome-present-state-test (OPT) model of reflective clinical reasoning. We discuss how this model serves as a conceptual framework for clinical reasoning. We compare and contrast the OPT model with the scientific method and the nursing process. We propose that the OPT model is the structure for clinical reasoning and that the knowledge classification systems are the content of clinical reasoning. In Chapter 4, we explore and explain why knowledge work is necessary for the advancement of clinical reasoning and the nursing profession. We describe several classification systems that support clinical reasoning. The role of knowledge classification systems in the development of the art and science of clinical reasoning is highlighted.

1

Quick Reference Table of Contents for Unit I

CHAPTER 1

The Art and Science of Clinical Reasoning: Nursing and Society

COMPETENCIES

After completing this chapter, the reader should be able to:

1. Define and explain why clinical reasoning is an essential nursing skill.

2. Explain how clinical reasoning supports the art and science of nursing.

3. Explain the importance of nursing to society.

4. Explain the four definitions of nursing described in the American Nurses Association (ANA) social policy statement.

5. Describe the American Association of Colleges of Nursing (AACN) vision statement on nursing education.

6. Discuss the Pew Health Professions Commission recommended competencies for health care providers.

7. Describe learning experiences needed to master the knowledge, skills and abilities defined by the social policy statement, the AACN vision document, and the Pew Health Professions Commission recommendations.

8. Explain the differences between an "action self" and a "reflective self."

9. Create an action plan to develop the reflective clinical reasoning required of a professional nurse.

INTRODUCTION

The contributions of nurses will be vital in meeting twenty-first-century health care challenges. In spite of advancements in disease prevention and health promotion, a need exists to educate people about healthy lifestyles and to provide care and counsel for people if and when they do become ill, disabled, or unable to care for themselves. Clinical reasoning is the heart of nursing. We define clinical reasoning as the reflective, concurrent, creative, and critical thinking embedded in nursing practice. Nurses develop clinical reasoning skills based on analysis and understanding of individual client stories. Each patient encounter presents opportunities to reason. Every time nurses reason about a client story, they add to their repertoire of understanding and the resources they have available to reason more effectively.

Albert Einstein (1927) once wrote, "If what is seen and experienced is portrayed in the language of logic, we are engaged in science. If it is communicated through forms whose connections are not accessible to the conscious mind, but are recognized intuitively as meaningful, then we are engaged in art" (p. 30). Nursing is both art and science. The *science* of nursing helps nurses analyze and evaluate data and make sound decisions concerning client care. The science of nursing is about logic. The *art* of nursing enables nurses to use intuition and experience to build meaningful relationships with clients and colleagues. The art of clinical reasoning is about connections that are recognized intuitively as meaningful. Nurses use knowledge from science as they work with and understand people's health care needs. This book is devoted to helping you understand how to reason more effectively about nursing care needs of people.

The art and science of nursing is grounded in a social contract and experiences with people in need. Understanding nursing in the larger context of society, what social forces are impinging on nursing, and what role you have to play in developing yourself as a professional is a place to begin.

THE ART AND SCIENCE OF NURSING IN THE CONTEXT OF SOCIAL POLICY

A profession is distinguished from other occupations by several criteria. A profession has an orientation toward service within the context of a code of ethics. A profession draws from a developed knowledge base and systematically uses theory to guide actions. In a profession there are standards of practice. A profession provides for the education and socialization of its members. A profession is autonomous and self-regulating. Professional self-regulation is the process by which nursing ensures that its members act in the public interest by providing a unique service that society has entrusted to them (ANA, 1995).

The social context of nursing is discussed in the ANA, social policy statement (ANA, 1980; 1995). "Nursing's Social Policy Statement is a document that nurses can use as a framework for understanding nursing's relationship with society and nursing's obligations to those who receive nursing care" (ANA, 1995, p. 1). The social policy statement provides a definition of nursing, explains the knowledge base for nursing practice, identifies the differences between basic and advanced nursing practice, and discusses the professional, legal, and self-regulated governance of nursing practice for the benefit of society. The social policy statement provides clues about the importance of thinking and reasoning to professional nursing practice.

In 1980, the social policy statement defined nursing as "the diagnosis and treatment of human responses to actual or potential health problems" (p. 6). This definition capitalized on advances nurses made in practice, research, and knowledge development. This definition represented a recognition of the crucial role thinking and diagnostic reasoning play in nursing practice. In 1995, the social policy statement was revised. Of particular interest to students are descriptions of nursing through time that are included in the revised document. Florence Nightingale (1859) defined nursing as those things nurses do "to put the client in the best condition for nature to act upon him" (p. 75). About a hundred years later, Virginia Henderson (1961) stated that the purpose of nursing is "to assist the individual, sick or well, in the performance of those activities contributing to health or its recovery (or to a peaceful death) that he would perform unaided if he had the necessary strength, will, or knowledge and to do this in such a way as to help him gain independence as rapidly as possible" (p. 5). Both definitions focused on nursing actions and what nurses do to promote health and healing.

As nurses strive to blend both the art and science of nursing, the social policy statement (1995) concludes that the essential features of contemporary nursing practice include:

1. attention to the full range of human experiences and responses to health and illness without restriction to a problem-focused orientation.
2. integration of objective data with knowledge gained from an understanding of the client's or group's subjective experience.
3. application of scientific knowledge to the processes of diagnosis and treatment.
4. provision of a caring relationship that facilitates health and healing (p. 6).

Each of the essential features requires clinical reasoning.

Nursing science involves the use of logic to understand and solve client problems. Research and the scientific method are the ways people use logic to generate knowledge that nurses use in client care. The scientific method is a problem-solving approach in which a problem is identified, possible solutions to the problem are hypothesized, and experiments are designed to test a solution to the problem. This is a step-by-step process guided by logic and reasoning that follows specific rules.

There are three kinds of nursing science: basic nursing science, applied nursing science, and practical science. Basic science refers to knowledge that is developed purely for the sake of knowing. This knowledge adds to our sense of understanding about people. It is generally understood that the knowledge may be useful someday. Applied nursing science is knowledge that is used in caring directly for clients. Both basic and applied science serve as the foundation for clinical reasoning. Johnson (1991) argues for a third type of science, which she calls practical science. Practical science combines the science and art of nursing. In nursing, more attention is often paid to the topic of science rather than art. However, "science alone will not solve all the problems of nursing" (Johnson, 1994, p. 1). Based on her review of the literature, Johnson (1994) discovered that art in nursing means

1. the ability to grasp meaning in client encounters
2. the ability to establish a meaningful connection with clients
3. the ability to skillfully perform nursing activities
4. the ability to rationally determine an appropriate course of action
5. the ability to morally conduct one's nursing practice

A challenge for future nurses is to figure out how to combine the science and art of nursing into a practical science. While the science of nursing is important, the art of nursing also deserves consideration.

A VISION FOR NURSING EDUCATION

The AACN is the national voice for university and four-year college education programs in nursing. In February 1998, the Association developed and published a vision statement about nursing education programs. The future of nursing education involves preparing students to manage and interpret data and evaluate nursing activities and interventions. Students need competencies in case management, financial management, health care policy, and economics. Research methods and knowledge of patient care outcomes and legislative initiatives are essentials for a nursing education program. Additionally, students need to learn skills of delegation and the ability to think and reason across a diversity of settings or contexts. Such a vision for nursing education requires development of strong clinical reasoning skills.

THE PEW HEALTH PROFESSIONS COMMISSION

The Pew Health Professions Commission evolved from a concern about the future of health in the United States. In order to influence the education and training of health care professionals, the Commission conducted surveys to determine what areas were important for professional training. The accompanying display lists the 16 competencies the Pew Commission deemed very important for health care providers to possess in the twenty-first century.

BOX 1-1   Pew Health Professions Competencies

1. Communicate effectively with clients and their families.
2. Problem-solve and think independently.
3. Make ethical decisions.
4. Provide health care services.
5. Pursue a lifetime of continuous learning.
6. Foster wellness and encourage preventive behaviors.
7. Involve clients and their families as partners in health care.
8. Work effectively in teams with other health care professionals.
9. Factor cost implications into decision making.
10. Ensure access to good health care for all segments of the population, including the least advantaged.
11. Manage large volumes of scientific and technical information.
12. Evaluate the appropriateness of complex and costly technology.
13. Respond to the increasing role in and scrutiny of your work by public, government, and health insurers.
14. Understand and respond to the diverse needs and values of different cultural or ethnic groups in the community.
15. Understand and support the important role that service agencies in the community play in meeting health needs.
16. Develop programs for aggregates and large populations.

From Shugars, DA, O'Neil, EH, Bader, JD, eds. *Health America: Practitioners for 2005,* an agenda for action for U.S. health professional schools. San Francisco, CA: The Pew Health Professions Commission, 1991. Reprinted with permission.

Out of the 16 competencies, five areas of professional training were identified across health care disciplines. The essential areas include (1) communicating with clients and families. Communication is both art and science. From your nursing studies you already realize the importance of communication skills in sending and receiving meaningful messages. (2) Involving clients and families as partners in their health care. Involving clients as partners in their health care is a function of values and beliefs you hold and communication styles you use. (3) Problem solving and thinking independently. Problem solving, thinking, and diagnosing are aspects of clinical reasoning. All health care professionals use a problem-solving model to diagnose and treat different aspects of individual, group, family, and/or community health care concerns. (4) Fostering wellness and encouraging preventive behavior. (5) Using ethical principals in decision making. Using these principles in decision making is a professional responsibility that is embedded in all health care practice.

BOX 1-2   Pew Essential Care Competencies

1. Communicate with clients and families
2. Involve clients and families as partners in health care
3. Problem-solve and think independently
4. Foster wellness and encourage preventive behavior
5. Use ethical principles in decision making

From Shugars, DA, O'Neil, EH, Bader, JD, eds. *Health America: Practitioners for 2005,* an agenda for action for U.S. health professional schools. San Francisco, CA: The Pew Health Professions Commission, 1991. Reprinted with permission.

Each of these competencies involves clinical reasoning. Clinical reasoning includes the activities of diagnosis, problem solving, outcome specification, and independent thinking. Ethics is a special kind of clinical reasoning that requires the science of logic and the art of valuing human experience. And of course, you need to be able to communicate effectively what and how you reason.

STOP AND THINK

How is your educational program organized to help you master the art and science of nursing? What learning experiences support the development of the AACN vision statement and the Pew Health Professions competencies?

The values and competencies deemed essential by the Pew Commission closely match definitions of nursing as art by Johnson (1991). Compare the essential competencies identified by the Pew Health Professions Commission with Johnson's notions of the art of nursing. Look at Table 1-1. The comparison between the Pew competencies and Johnson's description of art in nursing demonstrate how essential nurses will be in the twenty-first century. Blending art and science in nursing enables nurses of the future to meet the challenges set before all health care professionals.

REFLECTION AND RESPONSIBILITY

Up to this point in the chapter, we have examined social and political factors that are influencing the nursing profession. Success in nursing requires the development of

TABLE 1-1	**Nursing as Art Compared to Pew Health Professions Commission Competencies**
Pew ESSENTIAL COMPETENCIES	**NURSING AS ART**
1. Communicate with clients and families	1. Establish meaningful connections with clients
2. Involve clients and families as partners in health care	2. Grasp meaning in client encounters
3. Problem-solve and think independently	3. Rationally determine an appropriate course of action
4. Foster wellness and encourage preventive behavior	4. Skillfully perform nursing actions
5. Be sensitive to the ethics involved	5. Morally conduct one's nursing practice

an identity and commitment to the profession through the active use of an inquiring spirit. By asking, knowing, learning, and reflecting one comes to understand the art of nursing. What qualities do you think are essential to professional nursing practice? The AACN (1986) developed a statement about essentials of education for the professional nurse. Professional nurses value the following: altruism, equality, esthetics, freedom, human dignity, justice, and truth. In Table 1-2, qualities associated with essential nursing values are listed and defined. These values, attitudes, and personal qualities are expectations of professional nurses.

STOP AND THINK

Professional and personal values are important for success in nursing. Review the values of the professional nurse in the left-hand column of Table 1-2. Consider how these values support professional nursing practice. Review and reflect on the personal qualities in the right-hand column. Circle those qualities that best describe you with a black ink pen. Circle those qualities that you need or want to develop with a red pen. Stop and think about your answers to the following questions:

1. **Which qualities best describe you?**
2. **How did you develop these qualities?**
3. **What qualities do you not yet have?**
4. **What experiences do you need to acquire these qualities?**
5. **How do these qualities influence your thoughts, ideas, and feelings about nursing as art and science?**
6. **How are these qualities related to thinking and reasoning?**

TABLE 1-2 **Personal Qualities Checklist**	
VALUES OF THE PROFESSIONAL NURSE	**PERSONAL QUALITIES CHECKLIST**
ALTRUISM—concern for the welfare of others	Caring, Commitment, Compassion, Generosity, Perseverance
EQUALITY—having the same rights, privileges, or status	Acceptance, Assertiveness, Fairness, Self-Esteem, Tolerance
ESTHETICS—qualities of objects, events, and persons that provide satisfaction	Appreciation, Creativity, Imagination, Sensitivity
FREEDOM—capacity to exercise choice	Confidence, Hope, Independence, Openness, Self-Direction, Self-Discipline
HUMAN DIGNITY—inherent worth and uniqueness of an individual	Consideration, Empathy, Humaneness, Kindness, Respectfulness, Trust
JUSTICE—upholding moral and legal principles	Courage, Integrity, Morality, Objectivity
TRUTH—faithfulness to fact or reality	Accountability, Authenticity, Honesty, Inquisitiveness, Rationality, Reflectiveness

KNOWLEDGE WORK AND CLINICAL REASONING

Nurses are knowledge workers. Knowledge work is a prerequisite for effective clinical reasoning. In order to be a skilled nurse, you need to know the facts and use your knowledge. For example, normal blood pressure is 120/80. Deviation from this indicates a problem. If you didn't know what was normal, it would be difficult to make decisions about deviations from the norm. Knowledge workers rely on reasoning. Reasoning can be learned just as you learned how to use and work with knowledge in order to understand how the heart pumps blood. Clinical reasoning presupposes you have certain skills and attitudes. The prerequisite skills of clinical reasoning include activities associated with knowledge work: reading purposefully, memorizing, communicating ideas, understanding vocabulary, knowing the facts, putting facts together in meaningful ways, using facts, and deciding about the usefulness of facts for a particular situation. For example, in learning how the heart pumps blood, you needed to be able to read the text and memorize information about the heart. Then you learned the vocabulary, such as right ventricle, aorta, contraction, and electrical innervation. This same kind of learning process takes place as you learn to use clinical reasoning in your nursing practice.

CLINICAL REASONING AND ATTITUDE

In addition to knowledge work, clinical reasoning is also influenced by attitude. The prerequisite attitudes that you need for clinical reasoning are:

1. intent
2. reflection
3. curiosity
4. tolerance for ambiguity
5. self-confidence
6. professional motivation

Good thinking does not happen by accident. It happens by intent. With intent you have an idea about the end result of your actions and how you are going to organize your thinking to get there. Intent means that you have a deliberate plan of thinking and reason with a purpose in mind. The ability to have intentions requires that you understand the importance and differences between your "action self" and "reflective self." Reflection is the ability to see yourself thinking and doing. For some people, reflection is the ability to talk themselves through a situation. Whether you see yourself or talk to yourself, you really have two selves: an action self and a reflective self. The action self engages in activity while the reflective self watches or comments about the action self. (Refer to Figure 1-1.)

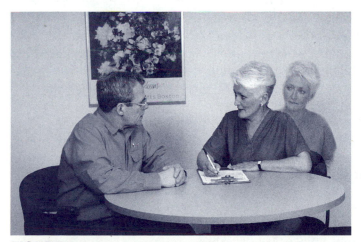

FIGURE 1-1 Clinical Reasoning Requires an Action Self and Reflective Self

People who have well-developed skills in clinical reasoning are able to have both selves functioning simultaneously. This text is designed to assist you with the development of your reflective self. Clinical reasoning develops best when you can reflect on past experiences. Clinical reasoning also develops when you are skilled enough to reflect while you are acting or doing. One way to develop expertise at reasoning is to look back on what you did and ask yourself questions about how and why you did what you did. Conducting a reflection check means you self-monitor your actions and thinking after an encounter with a client or think about your own thinking. Reflection is the way you become aware of what you are thinking (the content of your thinking), how you are thinking (the process of thinking), as well as why you are thinking (the premises of thinking).

Curiosity means you are eager to ask for and acquire information or knowledge. Isn't it interesting that the origin of this word is from the Latin word *cura,* which means to care (*American Heritage Dictionary,* 1985)? Reflection and curiosity go hand in hand. Nursing is curiosity (care) with a purpose. The greater your curiosity, the more tolerant of ambiguity you become. The more curious you are about the ways in which people think, act, and believe, the less likely you are to be judgmental. The greater your curiosity, the more compassion you are likely to possess.

Tolerance for ambiguity is the ability to feel comfortable when the situation is unclear and the outcome is undefined. Encounters with clients are often ambiguous. You don't know what the client is going to say or do, you don't know what is going to happen, and you don't know how you are going to react. Most people believe that situations have right answers. But right answers are seldom evident. For example, in some instances one is forced to choose between two goals. If you were forced to choose between truth or loyalty, which choice would you make? If you had to decide between a short-term or long-term gain for some project, which decision would you favor? The degree to which one can tolerate ambiguity is often a matter of self-confidence.

Self-confidence is believing in yourself, affirming yourself, and knowing that you are capable of thinking on your feet and responding appropriately. Part of self-confidence is knowing your strengths and weaknesses and obtaining the experiences required to develop the competencies you need. Self-confidence also involves knowing you possess the personal qualities and characteristics of a professional nurse.

Professional motivation is commitment to the vision, values, and mission of a profession. Taking on these values means that you will behave in a different way. For example, you will become your own judge. An individual's commitment to professional vision and mission requires skills in self-judgment. None of us is perfect and we all make mistakes in thinking and acting. A professional recognizes mistakes and then develops a plan of corrective action. You use your reflective self to make judgments about your professional behavior.

Now that you have been introduced to the prerequisite skills and attitudes of clinical reasoning, consider each factor. Answer the questions listed in the following "Stop and Think" associated with the skill and/or attitude, and then think about your answer to the questions posed.

STOP AND THINK

Knowledge
1. Do you know basic nursing facts, parameters, norms, and possible deviations from the norms?

Intention
1. Do you reason with purpose and intention?
2. Do you start with the end result in mind?
3. How do you organize your thinking to get to the end result?

Reflection
1. Are you able to see or describe yourself in action?

Curiosity
1. Do you eagerly search out new knowledge about a situation?
2. Are you comfortable asking questions?

Tolerance for ambiguity
1. How are you feeling about the situation?
2. Are you uncomfortable not knowing all the right answers?
3. How can ambiguity be useful?

Self-Confidence
1. What do you believe about your skills in this situation?
2. What are your professional motivations for seeking a nursing career?
3. How will you know you are the best nurse you can be?

CLIENT STORIES AND CLINICAL REASONING

Benner, Tanner, and Chesla (1996), in a book entitled *Expertise in Nursing Practice,* identified five attributes that are essential aspects to the art of nursing and the development of a practical science. First, nurses come to situations with a fundamental notion about what is good and right. There is a moral dimension to nursing. Second, expert nurses recognize patterns through experiences they have with clients. Third, expert nurses use their emotional involvement with clients to support their understandings, actions, and interventions. Fourth, expert nurses use their intuition formed from experience to guide their thinking and doing. Finally, expert nurses come to know clients through the stories that clients tell about their health care experiences. These stories provide information about the client that could not be obtained in any other way. The art of nursing is contained in stories clients share about their experiences and the stories nurses share about their clients.

STOP AND THINK

Think of a recent interaction with a client. Stop and think about your answers to the questions.

1. **Did the client have a story to tell?**
2. **What did you learn from listening to the client's story?**
3. **How do client stories influence you?**
4. **What were the moral or ethical dimensions to the client's story?**
5. **How did you respond to the story?**
6. **What emotional responses did the client's story invoke?**
7. **As you listened to the client story, did it remind you of any clients in your past?**
8. **Did the story have a recognizable pattern or meaning?**
9. **How might you use client stories as a guide for developing clinical reasoning skills?**

This book describes ways to think and reason about client stories. In the next few chapters we trace the history of the nursing process and explain new ways to think and reason. Nursing process is one way to think about client stories. We believe that the art and science of clinical reasoning has developed dramatically over the years. We believe the knowledge work that has been done in nursing requires new ways to think and reason about client stories. We hope to share our methods with you. Our goal is to help you develop the art and science of clinical reasoning.

SUMMARY

In this chapter, we have discussed social forces shaping nursing. Specifically, the AACN vision statement for nursing education offers a guide to the skills nurses will need in the future health care delivery context. The Pew Health Profession Commission has identified competencies that health care professionals of the future must have. Given nursing's contract with society, nurses fulfill an important role in promoting and maintaining the health of the nation. In fact, when one looks at the Pew competencies and the definitions of nursing as art, it is clear that the Pew Health Professions Commission competencies are consistent with nursing's mission, values, and vision. On a personal level, one needs to engage in values clarification regarding the characteristics essential for professional nursing practice. Nursing is about responsibility and reflection. On a professional level, one needs knowledge, intent, reflective capacity, curiosity, tolerance for ambiguity, self-confidence, and professional motivation. How you combine these values and characteristics will determine the balance of science and art in your nursing practice. One of the keys to success in developing clinical reasoning skills is the conscious development of an action self and a reflective self. In the next chapter, we will discuss the traditional paradigm of thinking in nursing—the nursing process. Nursing process provides a foundation for thinking in nursing. We believe nursing process is a foundation nursing skill that has changed over time. We suggest a transformation is needed in the traditional nursing process. Once the foundation is firm, nurses are able to build on this foundation and become more sophisticated in their thinking and reasoning.

KEY CONCEPTS

1. Clinical reasoning is the heart of nursing. There is an art and a science to clinical reasoning.
2. Clinical reasoning is the reflective, concurrent, creative, and critical thinking embedded in nursing practice.
3. The art and science of nursing are grounded in a social contract and experiences with people in need, visions of the profession, and competencies required of all health care providers..
4. Nursing as art involves establishing meaningful connections with clients, listening to and learning from client stories, and developing a rational, moral, skillful mode of practice.
5. In addition to knowledge work, clinical reasoning is influenced by attitude. The prerequisite attitudes that you need for clinical reasoning are

   - intent
   - reflection
   - curiosity
   - tolerance for ambiguity
   - self-confidence
   - professional motivation

6. Development of clinical reasoning skills involves responsibility and reflection. Reflection is becoming aware of an "action self" and a "reflecting self."
7. Listening to the stories clients tell is one way to capture the art of nursing while building reasoning skills. The stories people tell about their health care needs are opportunities for learning, practicing, reflecting and reasoning.

STUDY QUESTIONS AND ACTIVITIES

1. Read the ANA social policy statement and the AACN vision statement. How are these two documents alike and how are they different?
2. Review the essential values and characteristics from the 1986 AACN publication and identify what your current strengths and weaknesses are in reference to the values of the profession and your personal qualities checklist.

3. Review the skills and attitudes necessary for clinical reasoning. Identify the characteristics that are least developed in yourself and write a plan for strengthening those characteristics.

4. What is a metaphor, image, or object that best represents the relationship between art and science in nursing for you? Discuss your metaphors with classmates and nursing faculty.

5. Do you understand the differences between an "action self" and a "reflective self"? Create a personal plan of action for the development of these two self-parts. What do you need to develop the reflective self part of your professional self?

REFERENCES

American Association of Colleges of Nursing. (1998). *A vision of baccalaureate and graduate nursing education: The next decade*. Washington, DC: American Association of Colleges of Nursing.

American Association of Colleges of Nursing. (1986). *Essentials of college and university education for professional nurses*. Washington, DC: American Association of Colleges of Nursing.

American Heritage Dictionary. (1985). Boston, MA: Houghton-Mifflin.

American Nurses Association. (1995). *Nursing's social policy statement*. Washington, DC: American Nurses Association.

American Nurses Association. (1980). *Nursing: A social policy statement*. Washington, DC: American Nurses Association.

Benner, P. A., Tanner, C. A., & Chesla, C. A. (1996). *Expertise in nursing practice: Caring, clinical judgment, and ethics*. New York: Springer.

Einstein, A. (1995 [1927]). Letter to an editor of a German magazine. In Alan Eddington (Ed.), *Essential Einstein* (p. 30). Rohnert Park, CA: Pomegranate Art Books.

Henderson, V. (1961). *Basic principles of nursing care*. London: International Council of Nurses.

Johnson, J. (1994). A dialectical examination of nursing art. *Advances in Nursing Science, 17*(1), 1–14.

Johnson, J. (1991). Nursing science: Basic, applied, or practical? Implications for the art of nursing. *Advances in Nursing Science, 14*(1), 7–16.

Nightingale, F. (1859). *Notes on nursing: What it is and what it is not*. London: Harrison & Sons. (Facsimile ed. Philadelphia, PA: Lippincott, 1946).

Shugars, D. A., O'Neil, E. H., & Bader, J. D. (Eds.). (1991). *Healthy America: Practitioners for 2005, an agenda for action for U.S. health professional schools*. San Francisco, CA: The Pew Health Professions Commission.

CHAPTER 2

Nursing Process: Traditions and Transformations

COMPETENCIES

After completing this chapter, the reader should be able to:

1. Describe three generations and transformations of the nursing process.
2. Explain how the creation and development of nursing diagnoses and nursing knowledge classification work have influenced the traditional nursing process model.
3. Discuss advantages and disadvantages of the traditional nursing process model for contemporary nursing practice.
4. Describe the OPT model of clinical reasoning.
5. Compare and contrast the OPT model with the scientific method, problem solving, and the nursing process.

INTRODUCTION

As the health care industry shifts to an outcomes orientation, the nursing process needs modification. Reviewing the history of nursing process, one can pinpoint trends and transformations. These trends provide insights and an opportunity for discussion about modifications of the nursing process over time. Contemporary trends and forces suggest another transformation of the nursing process is needed. Teaching clinical reasoning over the past 10 years has provided us the opportunity to examine the nursing process and question how it works. We have identified three distinct generations of nursing process (Pesut & Herman, 1998). Each generation was influenced by the state of knowledge development and contemporary forces operative during its formation. A brief review of each generation is provided below.

FIRST-GENERATION NURSING PROCESS: PROBLEMS AND PROCESS—1950–1970

From the 1950s, the nursing process has provided structure for thinking in nursing. This process was designed to organize thinking so that patient problems nurses encountered could be anticipated and solved quickly. For example, Abdellah (1960) identified 21 nursing problems that were the focus of nursing care. This problem identification method stimulated educators to develop a problem-solving method grounded in assessment. A four-step process involving assessment, planning, intervention and evaluation (APIE) was developed and used (Yura & Walsh, 1988; National League for Nursing [NLN], 1992) Using the APIE model, nurses identified problems and procedures to deal with these problems.

This approach was valuable because it focused professional attention on the need to think before acting. As nurses gained experience with the nursing process, nursing knowledge was developed. Nursing education programs focused on problem- and solution-oriented nursing care. An assessment indicated a particular problem, and the solution or nursing care associated with the problem was determined and defined. Nursing actions, procedures, and interventions were developed and used in clinical settings.

Use of the four-step nursing process model helped practicing nurses zero in on specific problems. For example, care for appendectomy clients was related to a specific postoperative trajectory. On certain post-op days, specific patient progress was anticipated. Recovery was predictable. If there were deviations in the recovery, measures were instituted to get the patient back on track. The beginnings of critical paths were born in early nursing process, practice, and clinical contexts.

In some instances, problem identification and nursing solutions became routinized. The thinking involved in nursing care delivery was sometimes replaced by ritual and tradition or policies and procedures. Since the first generation of nursing process focused on nursing care needs of medical conditions, it is not surprising that many nursing problems and processes were related to pathophysiological conditions. As patterns of these problem solutions became apparent, a small group of nurses began to realize that there was a need to classify and standardize the nursing care problems that frequently required nursing attention.

These problems became the focus of the first Nursing Diagnosis Conference. In 1973, a group of nurses met in St. Louis, Missouri, and organized the first national conference for the classification of nursing diagnoses. The purpose of the conference was to initiate dialogue among practicing nurses about a standardized nomenclature that would describe commonly occurring clinical problems. Using both deductive and inductive reasoning processes, the participants arrived at some problem labels.

BOX 2-1 Diagnoses Approved at the First National Conference on the Classification of Nursing Diagnoses

Anxiety
Body fluids, depletion of
Bowel function, irregular
Cognitive functioning, alteration in level of
Comfort level, alterations in
Confusion
Digestion, impairment of
Faith, alterations in
Fear
Grieving
Lack of understanding
Manipulation
Mobility, impaired,
Motor incoordination
Noncompliance
Nutrition, alterations in
Regulatory function of skin, impairment of
Respiration, impairment of
Respiratory distress
Self-care activities, altered ability to perform
Self-concept, altered
Sensory disturbance
Sensory impairment
Significant others' adjustment to illness, impairment of
Skin integrity, impairment of
Sleep rest pattern, ineffective
Thought processes, impaired
Urinary elimination, impairment of
Verbal communication, impairment of

Reprinted with permission from Gebbie, K., & Lavin, M. (1975). *Classification of nursing diagnosis*. St. Louis, MO: Mosby. Reprinted with permission from the North American Nursing Diagnosis Association (NANDA) and Nursecom, Inc.

These diagnoses represented patterns of problems nurses recognized in their practice and that were influenced by nursing care within the independent domain of nursing practice. Prior to this time diagnosis was not a step in the nursing process. However, with the advent of these diagnoses it was important to modify the four-step nursing process. A new step called diagnosis was developed. The conceptualization of clinical diagnoses was derived from an analysis of an identified problem and etiologies that sustained the problem. (Refer to Figure 2-1.)

Note in this diagram that two levels of assessment are identified. First, there is an assessment of the specific problem. Second, there is an assessment of the etiology that sustains the problem. Note also that a relationship exists between the problem and etiology. The definition of etiology is important. Etiologies are not medical conditions, but those factors that nurses influence to bring about a change in a client's problem. Diagnosis of nursing problems shifted the nursing process model from one

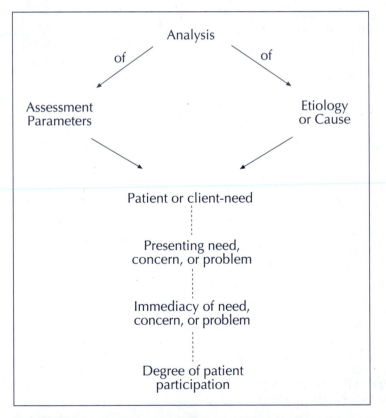

FIGURE 2-1 A Conceptualization of Nursing Diagnosis.
Reprinted with permission from Gebbie, K., & Lavin, M. (1975).
Classification of nursing diagnosis. St. Louis, MO: Mosby.
Reprinted with permission from the North American Nursing
Diagnosis Association (NANDA) and Nursecom, Inc.

of problem identification and solution finding to reasoning. Diagnostic reasoning involves the recognition of cues and analysis of data given specific clinical situations. The shift from problem identification and problem solving to diagnostic reasoning was a revolution in thinking that continues to have ripple effects in contemporary nursing practice. Studies on diagnostic reasoning and the critical thinking involved in nursing practice emerged (Kingten-Andrews, 1991; Miller & Malcolm, 1990; Jones & Brown, 1993; Facione & Facione, 1996). These studies were hallmarks and signs that a second generation of nursing process was beginning to evolve in the 1970s.

SECOND-GENERATION NURSING PROCESS: DIAGNOSIS AND REASONING—1970–1990

In 1973, the ANA published *Standards of Nursing Practice,* which established a five-step nursing process as a standard of care: assessment, diagnosis, planning, implementing, and evaluating. APIE was transformed into ADPIE—a five-step process that included the term "diagnosis." In the 1970s, the nursing diagnosis movement supported this transformation. Understanding the processes and products of diagnostic reasoning became a focus for clinical scholarship. Nursing diagnosis development generated research around the issues of diagnosis and diagnostic reasoning. Scholars (Carnevali, Mitchell, Woods, & Tanner, 1984; Gordon, 1982) began to tease apart the complexity involved in diagnostic reasoning. It became apparent that the nursing process required more than a problem–solution scenario. For example, *Nursing Diagnosis: Process and Application* by Marjory Gordon (1982) and *Diagnostic Reasoning in Nursing* by Carnevali, Mitchell, Woods, and Tanner (1984) described a way of thinking that offered an enhancement of the nursing process and was proposed to help nurses manage information and make decisions. These books defined diagnostic reasoning as a pattern of steps, including preencounter data, entry into the data search field, shaping direction of data gathering, cue clustering, determining diagnostic hypotheses, focusing the cue search, and testing hypotheses for "goodness of fit" in order to derive a diagnosis. The nature and type of terms now linked with thinking in nursing changed from problem identification to hypothesis formulation and testing. (See Figure 2-2.)

The diagnostic reasoning process explicated by Carnevali et al. (1984) and Gordon (1982) was a significant transformation. No longer was nursing process a logical, linear, stepwise problem-solving process. This second-generation model was influenced by theories and concepts of information processing and decision making.

As a result of developments in these areas, people began to question the usefulness of the traditional nursing process (McHugh, 1986). Others advocated the value of nursing process (Frisch, 1994). Advantages and disadvantages of the nursing process continue to be debated. Some of these advantages and disadvantages are listed in Table 2-1. Part of the debate involves confusion and discrepancy among the terms "diagnostic process," "decision making," "clinical reasoning," and "clinical judgment" (Kintgen-Andrews, 1991; Hamers, Abu-Saad, & Halfens, 1994).

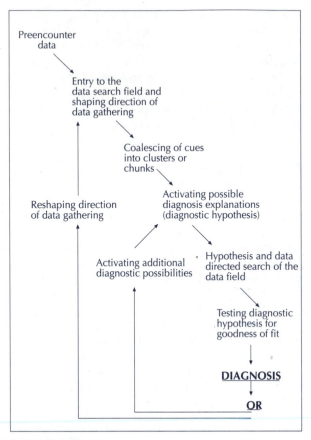

Preencounter data

Entry to the data search field and shaping direction of data gathering

Coalescing of cues into clusters or chunks

Reshaping direction of data gathering

Activating possible diagnosis explanations (diagnostic hypothesis)

Activating additional diagnostic possibilities

Hypothesis and data directed search of the data field

Testing diagnostic hypothesis for goodness of fit

DIAGNOSIS

OR

FIGURE 2-2   Diagnostic Reasoning Model. Reprinted with permission from Carnevali, D., Mitchell, P., Woods, N., & Tanner, C. (1984) *Diagnostic reasoning in nursing.* Philadelphia, PA: Lippincott.

STOP AND THINK

1. **Based on your recent clinical experiences, what do you think are the advantages and disadvantages of the nursing process?**
2. **Do you see nurses in practice using the nursing process as explicitly as you have learned it?**
3. **Do you agree or disagree that the nursing process is basically a problem-solving model?**
4. **If the nursing process did not exist, how might nurses reason about client care situations and nursing care requirements?**
5. **How does the five-step ADPIE model compare with the diagnostic reasoning model proposed by Carnevali, Mitchell, Woods, and Tanner (1984) in Figure 2-2?**

TABLE 2-1   Advantages and Disadvantages of the Traditional Nursing Process Model

ADVANTAGES	DISADVANTAGES
Model recognized by most nurses	Has become ritualized and routine
Long history and tradition in nursing	Difficult to apply new theories about thinking and reasoning
Structures content and process of thinking	Procedure-oriented
Stepwise, logical process	Outcome specification not explicit
Focuses on problem identification	Concurrent and creative thinking not emphasized
Problem identification leads to solution finding	Does not accommodate knowledge development
Care planning references are organized around nursing process	Deemphasizes reflective thinking
Provides structure and framework for teaching and learning nursing	Research supports variety of thinking processes
Professional standards of care are organized around the nursing process	Limits development of practice relevant theory

In the mid-1980s, Benner (1988) and Benner, Tanner, and Chelsa (1996) showed that novice and expert nurses used different thinking processes. Benner reframed and renamed many of the daily activities in which nurses are involved. Her studies indicated that expert nurses did not necessarily use the nursing process, but relied on experience and intuition and a combination of practical and academic intelligence. Exemplars illustrated how nurses coupled thinking with caring and ethics. The role of intuition and the person as the focus in reasoning about care needs was highlighted.

As the decade of the 1980s came to a close, the health industry shifted its attention from problems and diagnoses to specification and measurement of outcomes. Outcome specification became a central issue in health care reform. In fact, the most recent revision of the ANA social policy statement (1995) focused on outcomes and deemphasized problem-focused approaches to nursing care. Research on thinking and reasoning gave new insights into the nature of thinking and reasoning. These insights coupled with an interest in outcomes rather than problems set the stage for the next generation and transformation of the nursing process.

THIRD-GENERATION NURSING PROCESS: OUTCOME SPECIFICATION AND TESTING—1990–PRESENT

Contemporary nursing practice, with its focus on outcomes and complex analysis of multiple client conditions, requires critical thinking. Nursing diagnoses, interventions, and outcomes provide the clinical vocabulary for clinical reasoning in nursing. Developments in nursing intervention classification systems (McCloskey & Bulecheck, 1996; Maas, Johnson, & Moorhead, 1996) and classification of nursing-sensitive patient outcomes require new models of reasoning. Rather than "retro-fitting" new knowledge into an old process model, we believe there is a need for a completely different model of reasoning. In addition, there is a growing understanding of the role critical thinking plays in the reasoning process. Critical and creative thinking skills are essential to the development of nursing diagnoses, nursing knowledge, and practice-relevant theories.

We have developed a model to accommodate the changes in nursing process over time. We define clinical reasoning as reflective, concurrent, creative, and critical thinking embedded in nursing practice. Figure 2-3 illustrates the OPT model.

The OPT model provides a structure for the iterative reasoning necessary for contemporary nursing practice. Because we wanted to highlight the need for different processes involved in reasoning, the model flows from right to left. The OPT model is more comprehensive than the traditional nursing process. The model starts with a client's story.

The client-in-context story provides facts and cues that are linked in logical ways through cue logic. These linkages provide knowledge necessary to determine the frame, outcome state, present state, and test needed to determine if the outcome has been accomplished. Clinical decision making in this model is defined as choosing nursing actions to achieve the outcome. After nursing actions have been implemented or completed, a test is necessary. Testing is accomplished through the side-by-side comparison or juxtaposition of the outcome and present states. The juxtaposition creates a match or mismatch test condition. Concurrent judgment related to the match or mismatch determines the meaning of the test. The judgment may result in exiting the reasoning situation, altering decisions made about nursing actions, reformatting the test conditions, or reframing the situation. Reflection supports the entire clinical reasoning process.

COMPARING THE SCIENTIFIC METHOD, PROBLEM SOLVING, THE NURSING PROCESS, AND OPT

Table 2-2 illustrates a comparison among the OPT model, the nursing process, problem solving, and the scientific method.

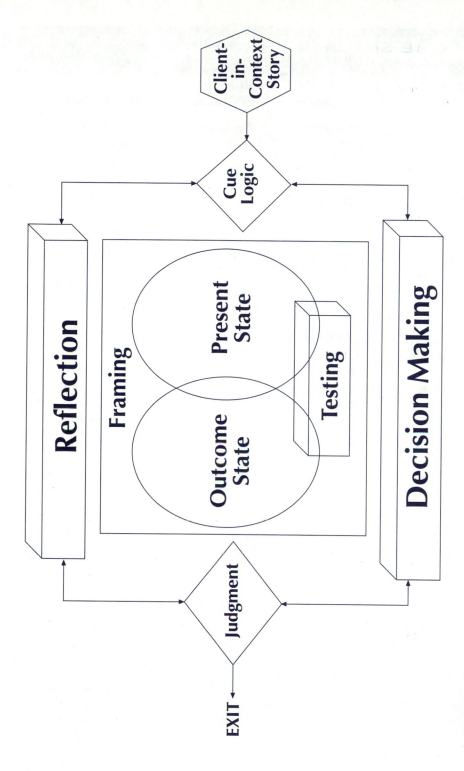

FIGURE 2-3 The Outcome-Present State-Test (OPT) Model of Reflective Clinical Reasoning

TABLE 2-2   A Comparison of the OPT Model, the Traditional Nursing Process, Problem Solving, and the Scientific Method

SCIENTIFIC METHOD	PROBLEM SOLVING	NURSING PROCESS	OPT MODEL
Recognizing problem	Encountering problem	Assessing	Client story Reflection Cue logic Framing
Collecting data	Collecting data		Determine present state Specifiy outcome Concurrently think about Frame
Formulating hypothesis	Identifying exact nature of problem	Formulating nursing diagnosis	Present state/ outcome Juxtaposition
Selecting plan for testing hypothesis	Determining plan of action	Planning	Make clinical decisions (interventions)
Testing hypothesis	Carrying out plan	Implementing	Act
Interpreting results	Evaluating plan in new situation	Evaluating	Test—identify gaps and evidence
Evaluating hypothesis			Make clinical judgments Reframe

As one examines the similarities and differences among the models, several observations unfold. First, all the models guide thinking in specific ways. All start with an organized assessment. All involve, in one way or another, diagnosis, evaluation, and judgment. There is a development and progression among the models, from identification of problems to framing of situations and contexts. The OPT model is unique, however, in terms of its explicit focus on the client's story as a way to frame relationships among contexts, present states, and desired outcomes. The OPT model underscores the fact that reasoning is concurrent and iterative, whereas the other models progress in stepwise fashion. In the OPT model, side-by-side comparisons of outcomes with present-state information about clients create test conditions about which judgments and conclusions are made given decisions and actions. The OPT model relies on higher-order thinking skills. In the OPT model there is a mechanism or point for terminating a reasoning task. Finally, the OPT model is more likely to accommodate present and future knowledge development activities in nursing and other disciplines. There are other differences to note. The nursing process is a linear process that focuses on problems and pieces of the story, specifically, who, what, and when. Evaluation is linked with goal achievement. The OPT model is more circular and fluid, exposes several problems, includes the "big picture," notes how the nurse can make a difference, and focuses on why and how one can act to promote or achieve the transition from a present to a desired state.

In the chapters that follow we will show how the OPT model is used as a basis for clinical reasoning. The beauty of the OPT model is that it can be used with different taxonomies that have different content. The underlying process, however, is the same. Knowledge work concerns bio-psycho-social facts. Nursing knowledge is contained in the North American Nursing Diagnosis Association (NANDA), Nursing Interventions Classification Project (NIC), Nursing Outcomes Classification Project (NOC), and Gordon nursing diagnoses taxonomies as well as the Omaha System. Knowledge of the *Diagnostic Statistical Manual-IV* (*DSM-IV*) is also useful to nurses.

We believe the OPT model will be most valuable once the work of NANDA, NIC, and NOC is more developed. Nursing diagnoses lend themselves to present-state conditions, nursing outcomes are likely to be desired states, and nursing interventions are likely to be decisions and actions that are used to bridge the gap between present and desired states. The OPT model provides a useful framework for all nurses, and creates an opportunity and means for blending the art and science of clinical reasoning in nursing.

SUMMARY

The traditional nursing process has changed over time. Three generations of the nursing process have been identified. The first generation (1950–1970) focused on problems and process. Over time nurses realized that the solutions to problems they encountered in practice needed identification and categorization. Nursing diagnoses were developed and retro-fitted into the nursing process. This development had profound implications for how nurses began to think and reason about nursing care situations The second generation (1970–1990) highlighted diagnosis and reasoning. Research in the area of diagnostic reasoning led to discoveries and insights about the advantages and disadvantages of the nursing process as model and method. Continued evolution and development of nursing knowledge classification systems as well as ongoing research into the dynamics of clinical reasoning has set the stage for another transformation of the nursing process. Organized knowledge in nursing practice provides the foundation for the clinical vocabulary necessary for clinical reasoning. The OPT model is a third-generation nursing process model that emphasizes reflection, outcome specification, and testing given a client's story. The OPT model builds on the heritage of the nursing process and is more responsive and relevant to contemporary nursing practice needs. Definitions and distinctions among the terms "clinical reasoning," "clinical decision making," and "clinical judgment" were made. In subsequent chapters we discuss how critical thinking and reflection as well as organized knowledge in nursing facilitate clinical reasoning.

KEY CONCEPTS

1. Nursing process started out as a four-step problem-solving model of assessment, planning, intervention, and evaluation.
2. Use of the nursing process over time led to the recognition of recurring nursing care problems called diagnoses.
3. Creation and development of nursing diagnoses required adding a step to the traditional nursing process model.
4. The advent of nursing diagnoses created a shift in thinking from problem solving to diagnostic reasoning.
5. A focus on diagnostic reasoning has heightened the influence thinking has on nursing practice.
6. Traditional nursing process has both strengths and weaknesses. The traditional nursing process is a useful foundation on which to build more complex thinking skills involved in the clinical reasoning process.
7. The OPT model provides a structure for a systems-based reasoning process. The OPT model is a third-generation nursing process model that provides the structure and process for contemporary nursing practice demands.

STUDY QUESTIONS AND ACTIVITIES

1. In your own words describe the relationship between problem solving and the nursing process.
2. Find and read a copy of the proceedings from the first North American Nursing Diagnosis Conference. If you had attended the conference, what do you imagine your reactions would be if you were an experienced nurse or student at the time?
3. Read or review the NANDA Conference proceedings from over the past 10 years. What themes are apparent? What issues interest you? Have these issues been resolved?
4. Organize a debate about the advantages and disadvantages of the nursing process. Create an argument for why it should stay the same and why it is the best method for organizing thinking in nursing practice.

5. What is your position on the development and testing of nursing diagnoses? Explain the pros and cons associated with the development of nursing diagnoses, nursing interventions and nursing outcomes.

REFERENCES

Abdellah, F. G. (1960). *Patient centered approaches to nursing.* New York: Macmillan.

American Nurses Association. (1995). Nursing's social policy statement. Washington, DC: American Nurses Association.

American Nurses Association. (1973). *Standards of nursing practice.* Kansas City, MO: American Nurses Association.

Benner, P. (1988). *From novice to expert.* Menlo Park, CA: Addison-Wesley.

Benner, P., Tanner, C., & Chesla, C. (1996). *Expertise in nursing practice.* New York: Springer.

Bowles, K., & Naylor, M. (1996). Nursing intervention classification systems. *Image: Journal of Nursing Scholarship, 28*(4), 303–308.

Carnevali, D., Mitchell, P., Woods, N., & Tanner, C. (1984). *Diagnostic reasoning in nursing.* Philadelphia, PA: Lippincott.

Delphi Report—Critical Thinking: A statement of expert consensus for purposes of educational assessment and instruction (1990). Research findings and recommendations prepared for The American Philosophical Association. P. Facione, Project Director, ERIC Doc. No. ED 315-42.

Facione, N. C., & Facione, P. A. (1996). Externalizing the critical thinking in knowledge development and clinical judgment. *Nursing Outlook, 44*(3), 129–136.

Flavell, J. (1979). Metacognitive and cognitive monitoring: A new era of cognitive-developmental inquiry. *American Psychologist, 34,* 906–911.

Fowler, L. (1997). Clinical reasoning strategies used during care planning. *Clinical Nursing Research, 4*(6), 349–361.

Frisch, N. (1994). Editorial: The nursing process revisited. *Nursing Diagnosis, 5*(2), 51.

Gebbie, K. M., & Lavin, M. A. (1975). *Classification of nursing diagnoses: Proceedings of the first national conference.* St. Louis, MO: Mosby.

Gordon, M. (1982). *Nursing diagnosis.* New York: McGraw-Hill.

Hall, L. (1955). Quality of nursing care. *Public health news.* Newark, NJ: State Department of Health.

Hamers, J., Abu-Saad, H., & Halfens, R. (1994). Diagnostic process and decision-making in nursing: A literature review. *Journal of Professional Nursing, 10*(3), 154–163.

Herman, J. A., Pesut, D. J., & Conard, L. (1994). Using metacognitive skills: The quality audit. *Nursing Diagnosis, 5*(2), 56–64.

Jones, S. A., & Brown, L. N. (1993). Alternative views on defining critical thinking through the nursing process. *Holistic Nursing Practice, 7*(3), 71–75.

Kintgen-Andrews, J. (1991). Critical thinking and nursing education: Perplexities and insights. *Journal of Nursing Education, 7*(4), 152–157.

Kitchener, K. (1983). Cognition, metacognition, and epistemic cognition: A three level model of cognitive processing. *Human Development, 26,* 222–232.

Maas, M., Johnson, M., & Moorhead, S. (1996). Classifying nursing sensitive patient outcomes. *Image: Journal of Nursing Scholarship, 28*(4), 295–301.

McCloskey, J., & Bulechek, G. (1996). *Nursing interventions classification.* St. Louis, MO: Mosby-Year Book.

McHugh, M. (1986). Nursing process: Musings on the method. *Holistic Nursing Practice, 1*(1), 21–28.

Miller, M. A., & Malcolm, N. S. (1990). Critical thinking in the nursing curriculum. *Nursing Health Care, 11*(2), 67–73.

National League for Nursing. Council for baccalaureate and higher degree programs. (1992). *Criteria for the evaluation of baccalaureate and higher degree programs in nursing* (6th ed.). NLN Publication No. 15-1252. New York: National League for Nursing.

Pesut, D., Herman, J. (1998). OPT: Transformation of nursing process for contemporary practice. *Nursing Outlook, 46*(1), 29–36.

Pesut, D., & Herman, J. A. (1992). Metacognitive skills in diagnostic reasoning. *Nursing Diagnosis, 3*(4), 148–154.

Pesut, D., Herman, J., & Fowler, L. (1997). Toward a revolution in thinking: The OPT model of clinical reasoning. In: J. McCloskey & H. Grace (Eds.), *Current issues in nursing* (5th ed., pp. 88–92). St. Louis, MO: Mosby.

Senge, P. (1990). *The fifth discipline.* New York: Doubleday.

Sternberg, R. (1988). *The triarchic mind.* New York: Viking.

Worrell, P. (1990). Metacognition: Implications for instruction in nursing education. *Journal of Nursing Education 29,* 170–175.

Yura, H., & Walsh, M. B. (1988). *The nursing process: Assessment, planning, implementation and evaluation* (5th ed.). Norwalk, CT: Appleton & Lange.

CHAPTER **3**

The OPT Model of Clinical Reasoning

COMPETENCIES

After completing this chapter, the reader should be able to:

1. Explain how the OPT model shifts the traditional nursing process.
2. Define terms associated with critical thinking.
3. Define terms associated with reflective clinical reasoning.
4. Define terms associated with thinking strategies that support clinical reasoning.
5. Define terms associated with the OPT model of clinical reasoning.
6. Discuss how the OPT model facilitates clinical reasoning.

INTRODUCTION

We believe the OPT model provides a framework that addresses the current outcome-focused agenda of the health care industry, fosters higher-order thinking skills, and accommodates present and future knowledge development activities in nursing. The model also complements the art of nursing because an essential part of the model involves listening and grasping the meaning in a client encounter. Using the client's story to "frame" or derive the meaning and significant issues helps structure and guide the thinking. We concluded the previous chapter with a definition of clinical reasoning. For our purposes clinical reasoning is the reflective, concurrent, creative, and critical thinking processes nurses use in practice to understand and frame client stories as well as organize nursing actions to achieve desired outcomes.

Clinical decision making in the OPT model is the process of choosing nursing actions and interventions. Clinical judgment in the OPT model is the process of attributing meaning to evidence or results of tests that are side-by-side comparisons of present-state data at any point in time with outcome criteria. The model shifts thinking from a problem orientation to an outcome orientation.

STOP AND THINK

Think back to a recent clinical decision you made. How, specifically, did you go about making that decision? Did you gather all the information about the client, organize that information into a problem list, develop the goals for the client, select a group of interventions, implement the interventions, and evaluate the effectiveness? Did you organize your care around the problem, or did you intervene to achieve an outcome? Were your actions really guided by the nursing process? Were you aware of how you were thinking? Did a theory guide your practice? How did you evaluate your own thinking in this instance?

ACADEMIC AND PRACTICAL INTELLIGENCE

Students say that nursing care plans in the hospital are not like the ones that teachers require. Nursing students comment that demands of the "real world' do not call for elaborate nursing care plans. In fact, in many institutions nursing care plans have been replaced by checklists, care maps, and critical pathways. These critical paths are road maps that help determine the progress a client is or is not making along a predetermined trajectory. Maps and pathways do not relieve nurses from the responsibility of making judgments about client care. What happens, for instance, if a client deviates from the path? How does one reason about deviations from the norm? Clinical reasoning is required when there is no standard plan or when clients deviate from the expected trajectory. Under these circumstances, professional nurses draw on past experiences, use accumulated knowledge, analyze existing data, and formulate a plan of care to remedy the situation.

SHIFTING FROM PROBLEMS TO OUTCOMES

A major focus of the change in health care is interest in identification and achievement of client health outcomes. To function effectively in this arena, nurses need outcome specification skills. The nursing process model and many nursing diagnoses are problem-focused. Clinical reasoning that focuses on outcomes is more valuable and cost-effective than clinical reasoning that focuses on problems. The OPT model organizes thinking to focus on outcomes.

THE OPT MODEL OF CLINICAL REASONING

The OPT model was derived and developed from the test-operate-test-exit (TOTE) model (Miller, Galanter, & Pribram ,1960). Dilts, Epstein, and Dilts (1991) used the TOTE model to explain creative thinking and the management of innovations. Using the structure of the TOTE model, we crafted the OPT model to represent the dynamic, concurrent, critical, and creative thinking nurses engage in as they reason about clinical situations. Reflection, framing, cue logic, testing, decision making, and judgment are essential processes contained within the OPT model. The model underscores the importance of framing and focusing on outcomes. If you are new to nursing, you will have to learn this model step by step. If you are an expert nurse, you are likely to feel a sense of familiarity with the model because it "unpacks" the essential strategies used by expert nurses.

Learning something new is sometimes uncomfortable. But little by little learning takes place. Remember when you were learning to read? There was a sequence of developmental steps along the way. First, you mastered the alphabet. Once you knew the letters, you learned that the letters could be combined into words. Words were used to create sentences. Sentences linked together created paragraphs. Paragraphs are components of stories, essays, and arguments. There are multitudinous ways to combine words to express your thoughts, feelings, emotions, and actions. Like learning the alphabet, we want to introduce you to the parts or ABCs of the OPT model. The OPT model is represented in Figure 3-1. Look at the model periodically as you read the following description and explanation.

A major difference between the OPT model and previous models is the emphasis on framing a situation based on the story of the client. Over the years we witnessed the following scenario. Students receive clinical assignments that often consist of a person's name and medical diagnosis. Students then go to the library and learn everything possible about the pathophysiology of the medical condition and the nursing care consequences of the condition. The students consult many of the nursing texts for relevant nursing diagnoses and care plans. Students return with drafted care plans, ready to fill in the blanks. To our shock and disbelief many students had care plans complete before ever seeing, hearing, touching, talking to, or listening to a client's story! While efficient, such an approach is clinically negligent. Client stories provide essential information and insights about the types and kinds of nursing care clients need.

Client Stories and Framing

A client's story provides important information regarding the context and major issues for clinical reasoning. Listening to clients, connecting with them in meaningful ways,

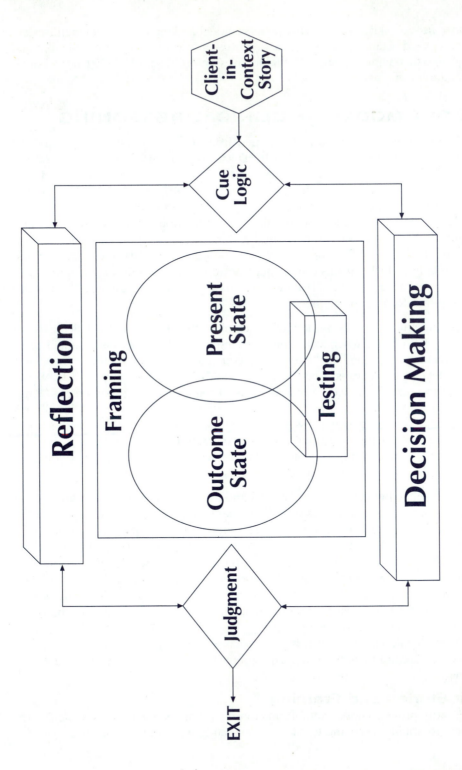

FIGURE 3-1 The OPT Model of Reflective Clinical Reasoning

attributing meaning to their stories, and getting the facts about their situation is the art of nursing. Stories are key element of clinical reasoning. How you "frame" a story has implications for how you reason. Consider the example in "Stop and Think."

STOP AND THINK

Mr. George Appleton is a 99-year-old gentleman in the intensive care unit (ICU) with a diagnosis of end-stage renal disease. If you "frame' this situation as "need to keep Mr. Appleton alive and maintain urinary output at 30 cc hour," how does such a frame guide and direct your thinking and doing? Would your thinking and doing be different if the "frame" or lens you used to view this situation involved "promoting a peaceful death"? How would thinking and doing be different given these two different perceptual positions?

We constantly frame situations. Frames are mental models or perceptual positions about issues, events, and meanings. Peter Senge (1990) discusses mental models in his book, *The Fifth Discipline*. Mental models determine how we make sense of the world and take action. Senge writes: "Mental models can be simple generalizations such as 'people are untrustworthy' or they can be complex theories, such as assumptions about why members of my family interact as they do. But what is most important to grasp is that mental models are active—they shape how we act. If we believe people are untrustworthy, we act differently from the way we would if we believed they were trustworthy. If I believe that my son lacks self-confidence and my daughter is highly aggressive, I will continually intervene in their exchanges to prevent her from damaging his ego" (1990, p. 175).

Frames are mental models that influence and guide our perception and behavior. Becoming aware of mental models in regard to client stories is an important aspect of clinical reasoning. Fairhurst and Sarr (1996) in their book *The Art of Framing* write, "to hold the frame of a subject is to choose one particular meaning or set of meanings over another" (p. 21). Here are some other observations they have about the importance of framing:

- Framing is a way to manage meaning. It involves the selection and highlighting of one or more aspects of a subject while excluding others.

- Framing involves the use of language, thought, and forethought. Language helps focus, classify, remember, and understand one thing in terms of another.

- Framing increases our chances of implementing goals and getting people's agreement, once the right frames are in place, the right behavior follows.

- Framing requires initiative, which includes both a clarity of purpose and a thorough understanding of those for whom we are managing meaning.

- Opportunities for framing occur with every communication.

- Our values play an important role in the kind of framing that we do and in the way that we and our frames are perceived (pp. 2–4).

Think of frames as different types of camera lenses. A wide-angle lens frames a scene much differently than a close-up zoom lens. Becoming aware of mental models and the frames we put on client stories is crucial to successful clinical reasoning. We become aware of frames through stories clients share with us and the meanings we attribute to those stories. The meaning we attribute to client stories is often translated into shorthand themes. For example, after listening to someone's story we might conclude the main issue is about frustration, anxiety, or coping. Framing is understandable once we take time to reflect on what we see, hear, know, and feel in the clinical moment. Framing is like the headline or caption of a client's situation or story. Critical thinking skills, reflective reasoning, and specific thinking strategies support framing and reasoning.

CRITICAL THINKING, REFLECTIVE REASONING, AND THINKING STRATEGIES

There is great interest today in critical thinking skills. Critical thinking skills support reflective clinical reasoning. Reflective clinical reasoning is supported by specific thinking strategies. Consider both the model in Figure 3-1 and Table 3-1 that illustrate how critical thinking skills are related to reflective clinical reasoning and how specific thinking strategies can be used to support this reflective reasoning.

At the heart of any reasoning model is the practitioner's ability to engage in reflective critical thinking. Facione and Facione (1996) define critical thinking as purposeful self-regulatory judgment that gives reasoned consideration to evidence, context, conceptualizations, methods, and criteria. Critical thinking includes many skills. Major skills are interpretation, analysis, evaluation, inference, explanation, and self-regulation. Terms associated with reflective clinical reasoning will be defined as we describe the model. In Table 3-1 we have mapped out relationships and associations among critical thinking skills and reflective clinical reasoning using the OPT model. Table 3-2 defines the thinking strategies that support both the reasoning model and critical thinking. We have also identified some specific thinking strategies we believe support the acquisition of clinical reasoning skills. Reflective clinical reasoning is a specific instance of critical thinking in nursing practice. Clinical reasoning is supported by higher-order critical thinking skills and lower-order thinking strategies. Thinking strategies help nurses engage in reflective clinical reasoning.

In the OPT model, reflection is a component of executive thinking processes and consists of critical, creative, and concurrent thinking. Reflection is the process of observing yourself think while simultaneously thinking about client situations. The goal of reflection is to achieve the best possible thought processes. The greater the reflection, the higher the quality of care delivered. Reflection involves use of the skills

TABLE 3-1 Relationships among Thinking Strategies, Reflective Clinical Reasoning, and Critical Thinking Skills

CRITICAL THINKING SKILLS	REFLECTIVE CLINICAL REASONING	THINKING STRATEGIES
Interpretation categorize decode sentences clarify meaning	**Knowledge work and** clinical vocabulary classification systems (e.g., NANDA, Gordon, Omaha, DSM-IV, NIC)	reading memorizing drilling writing reviewing research practicing
Analysis examine ideas identify arguments analyze arguments	**Cue logic** cue connection induction deduction retroduction	self-talk schema search prototype identification hypothesizing
Inference query evidence conjecture alternatives draw conclusions	**Framing** cue connection scenario development outcome specification test creation	schema search prototype identification hypothesizing if–then thinking
Explanation state results justify procedures present arguments	**Decision making** interventions alternatives consequences	schema search prototype identification comparative analysis if–then thinking
Evaluation assess claims assess arguments	**Testing** conduct test evaluate	juxtaposing comparative analysis reflexive comparison
Self-regulation self-examination self-correction	**Judgment** attribute meaning to the test outcome frame new situation create new test	reframing self-talk cue logic reflection check

TABLE 3-2 Thinking Strategies and Definitions	
THINKING STRATEGY	**DEFINITION**
Knowledge Work	Active use of reading, memorizing, drilling, writing, reviewing research, and practicing to learn clinical vocabulary
Self-Talk	Expressing one's thoughts to one's self
Schema Search	Accessing general and/or specific patterns of past experiences that might apply to the current situation
Prototype Identification	Using a model case as a reference point for comparative analysis
Hypothesizing	Determining an explanation that accounts for a set of facts that can be tested by further investigation
If–Then Thinking	Linking ideas and consequences together in a logical sequence
Comparative Analysis	Considering the strengths and weaknesses of competing alternatives
Juxtaposing	Putting the present state condition next to the outcome state in a side-by-side contrast
Reflexive Comparison	Constantly comparing the client's state from time of observation to time of observation
Reframing	Attributing a different meaning to the content or context of a situation based on tests, decisions, or judgments
Reflection Check	Self-examination and self-correction of critical thinking skills and thinking strategies that support clinical reasoning

of monitoring, analyzing, predicting, planning, evaluating, and revising. Critical thinking consists of developing the skills of interpretation, analysis, inference, explanation, evaluation, and self-regulation as well as the subskills listed in Tables 3-1 and 3-2 (Facione & Facione, 1996).

Knowledge Work and Clinical Vocabulary

One needs to be a knowledge worker and have a clinical vocabulary with which to reason. A clinical vocabulary helps one interpret, categorize, and decode sentences and clarify meanings. The clinical vocabulary for clinical reasoning in nursing consists of those knowledge classification systems that store nursing knowledge. The thinking strategies one uses to get this knowledge are such techniques as reading, memorizing, drilling, writing, reviewing research, and practicing. For example, it is easier to reason if you know "by heart" NANDA (1996) nursing diagnoses.

Framing and Inference

Framing involves thinking about the client's story. Framing includes distinguishing between the central issue or problem and peripheral problems. In terms of clinical reasoning, framing is the process of creating meaning out of the client's story in order to establish starting and stopping points for your reasoning efforts. Think of framing as the backdrop or scenery of a stage play. As the scenery and contexts change so do the actions and behavior of the actors. The background and context influence the action and events. Framing is one of the unique aspects of the OPT model. Framing a problem, event, or situation is like having a lens through which we view the client's story. The frame interacts with and provides the organizing structure for establishing the present state and outcome state desired. In order to frame a situation, you need to take into account the client's story and develop a scenario or projected chain of events associated with the story. In order to frame a situation, you need to take the long view or use "balcony thinking" (Senge, 1994). In other words, what are the central issues in the story? Ask yourself the questions, "What and how am I thinking about this story?" "What lens have I used to view this situation?" Framing is best accomplished by your reflective self. Of course, how you frame or attribute meaning to a situation depends on how you organize the data or cues associated with the story. So, framing depends on your use of cue logic. Cue logic is an important part of the OPT model.

Cue Logic

Cue logic is the deliberate structuring of client-in-context data to discern the meaning for nursing care. Cue logic can be inductive, deductive, or dialectic. Remember, induction involves reasoning from specific cues toward a general judgment. For example, redness in a wound with the presence of pus and an increased temperature leads one to conclude that the wound is infected. Deduction involves reasoning from a general premise toward a conclusion. For example, if infection is present, then antibiotics are likely to be an effective treatment. Dialectic thinking considers both the deductive and inductive aspects of a situation in terms of an open system subject to feedback and change. Once a client with an infected wound has been on antibiotics for a while, then the temperature should return to normal and redness should decrease.

Clinical evidence about the client-in-context is processed according to a nurse's cue logic. Cue logic contributes information that helps structure, or frame a situation. Cue logic is supported by the thinking strategies of self-talk—expressing one's thoughts to one's self. Cue logic is also influenced by memories or schema searches. In a schema search you retrieve general and/or specific patterns of past experiences that might apply to the current situation. Use of prototypes is another way to help you think about a situation. Prototypes are model cases that serve as reference points.

Hypothesizing means determining an explanation that accounts for a set of facts and that can be tested by further investigation.

Consider the example of the infected wound. Identification of pus and an increase in temperature leads one to ask the question about infection. Since past experience influences thinking, perhaps experience with an infected wound influences reasoning. Textbook descriptions of wound infections are helpful in using cue logic about this problem. Once treatment is initiated one can compare the healing wound with a memory of what it looked like with the infection present. This comparison is a test. The differences between the infected and healing wound create a contrast and provide evidence that means the wound is or is not healing.

Cue logic is useful in making sense of the client's story and framing the nursing care needs given the story and context in which one is working. Cue logic and framing go hand in hand and oscillate back and forth between figure and ground. For example, have you seen those perceptual illusions that depict an old woman or young woman? The stimuli are the same but your perception and frame differ depending on your glance.

Framing is the process of attributing meaning to connections among cues in order to establish the structure for testing achievement of outcomes. Framing is accomplished with the support of a schema search—accessing general and/or specific patterns of past experiences that might apply to the current situation; prototype identification—using a model case as a reference point for comparative analysis; and hypothesizing—determining an explanation that accounts for a set of facts and that can be tested by further investigation. If–then thinking is a thinking strategy that involves future time projection that considers the consequences of specific actions. It will make a differences how you frame the facts about the wound discussed in the earlier example. If the situation is framed as an infection, how does that guide your thinking? If the situation is framed as wound management, how does that influence thinking? If the situation is framed as wound healing, how does this influence thinking? If one frames the issue around elevated temperature, how does this frame influence thinking and doing? If the patient is a diabetic and the wound is on a lower extremity, how does the framing of the problem shift? The fact is that one must consider all of these possibilities at the same time. That is concurrent thinking.

With the frame as the background what now comes to the foreground is the development of a present state and outcome state comparison. The present state (P) is a description of the client-in-context, or the initial condition of the client. The present state, which changes over time as a result of nursing actions, is derived from cue logic and defined by standardized taxonomic terms. Using the example of the wound, the present state is impaired skin integrity. Outcomes (O) are desired or end states that result from nursing care. Outcome states are the desired conditions of the client derived from the frame and initial present-state data as well as criteria that define the desired condition. In the wound example, a desired outcome is healing, with integrity of skin and no infection.

Given the frame of a situation, nurses use outcome-focused thinking (Pesut, 1989) to create outcomes derived from present-state data. Once an outcome is derived, a side-by-side comparison of present to desired state is made. Juxtaposing is the side-by-side comparison of specified outcome state criteria with present-state data. Foreground issues of juxtaposed present and desired states emerge from background issues of "framing." The context is thus incorporated and supports the contrast of the juxtaposed present state/desired comparison. This side-by-side comparison creates a test (T). A test is the process of juxtaposing the present state and outcome state and evaluating the gap between the two states. During testing the nurse determines how well the gap has been filled. Nurses choose interventions to bring clients and families closer to desired states based on present-state data. Testing is accomplished through the use and application of comparative analysis and reflexive comparison, which is the process of making a judgment about the state of a situation after gauging the presence or absence of some quality against a standard using the current case as a reference criterion (Fowler, 1994). For example, how does the wound look one week after treatment? Conclusions related to tests are the bases of clinical judgments.

DECISION MAKING

Clinical decision making is the selection of interventions and actions that move clients from a presenting state to a specified or desired outcome state. Decision making in this model is when one considers and selects interventions from a repertoire of actions that facilitate the achievement of a desired outcome state. Decision making is supported through the use and application of schema searches and prototype identification. Comparative analysis is the process of considering the strengths and weaknesses of competing alternatives. If–then thinking also supports decision making.

Judgment is the process of drawing conclusions based on the findings from the test of the comparison of present state to a specified outcome state. Once judgments of present state closely match the desired outcomes (e.g., the wound is healed), the nurse can reason about other things. If a match or test is unsatisfactory (infection still present), reflection activates critical, creative, concurrent thinking and decision making. In terms of judgments, three conclusions are possible:

1. a perfect match between outcome state and present state (the wound is healed)
2. a partial match of outcome state with present state (wound healing is progressing but is not complete)
3. no match between outcome and present state (the wound is not healed and looks worse).

Judgments result in reflection and conclusions about actions to take based on the degree of match between the client's present state and the outcome state. Thinking strategies that support judgment are reframing or attributing a different meaning to the facts or evidence at hand. Finally, a reflection about the entire process results in self-correction, and the development of a schema or memory for future use!

CASE STUDY: MS. CORA JAMES' STORY

Let's look at the following case study and see if you can apply the OPT model of clinical reasoning. Given the facts, how do you use cue logic, framing, testing, decision making, and judgment to determine nursing care in this situation?

Ms. Cora James is a 65-year-old grandmother living in substandard housing. She presents in the clinic with the following cues: progressive weight loss; productive cough; oral temperature 101 degrees; weight 106 pounds; extended family living in substandard housing; and five young children at risk for infectious diseases, two childbearing daughters, and an alcoholic son living with her. Her records show that she is supposed to be receiving medication for tuberculosis.

How would you approach this case using the nursing process? The traditional nursing process is valuable in that it makes explicit the problem and the present situation. For example, one could focus on symptoms of pulmonary infection, possible noncompliance with medication regimen, weight loss, family at risk for contacting and spreading TB, and questionable availability of resources. How do the facts help "frame" the situation?

Clinically, focusing on the present state or presenting problems does not provide *explicit* direction for action. Once outcomes are specified, the path of action is clear and the tests of achievement are *explicit*. Transforming problems into outcomes involves thinking beyond the present to the end results of action. This outcome specification step, underdeveloped in the nursing process, is a primary focus in the OPT model. Also, framing is key in setting directions and priorities.

Consider use of the OPT model and monitor your thinking processes as you decide how to approach the Ms. James' case study. What is her story? How will you frame this situation? Depending on how you frame the situation, several outcomes are important in this case. Possible outcomes include: infection clear, afebrile, taking medication as prescribed, adequate resources, transportation for follow-up, and screening and treatment of family members. Focusing on the outcome of taking medication as prescribed, the nurse juxtaposes the present state with the outcome state and uses decision making to generate possible actions.

For example, the nurse might determine (frame the situation) that the client does not have resources to obtain the medication. Are Ms. James' problems best framed as a resource issue? Then, the nurse could implement a plan to obtain medication for the client using social service resources. Another possibility is that the client is unable to remember to take medication. Perhaps the issue is more likely framed as one of self-care deficit. The nurse could develop a plan for a family member to manage administration of the medication. The test comes when the nurse compares the present state to the desired outcome. If the present state on the next visit reveals that a family member obtained medication from social services and reported administering all medicines as prescribed, the outcome of taking medication as prescribed would be achieved. The nurse can go on to another reasoning task, and add this experiment to her repertoire of clinical reasoning schemas.

Based on this example, OPT was made explicit. Through the use of reflection, cue logic, framing, and clinical decision making, testing revealed a match and a judgment was made that the desired outcome was achieved. The OPT model makes more explicit the kind of reflective thinking strategies that are involved in clinical reasoning given a client's story. Learning how to use the clinical vocabulary of nursing knowledge contained in classification systems is our next learning challenge.

SUMMARY

We have proposed a new model of clinical reasoning—the OPT model. We believe the OPT model differs considerably from the traditional nursing process. The model has several strengths. First, it is built on a foundation of reflective judgment and is derived from empirical data. Second, the OPT model honors the holistic nature of nursing. Third, the OPT model approaches client situations in terms of outcomes. Fourth, the model identifies the thinking skills and strategies involved in making clinical decisions and judgments. Finally, the model can be used with several taxonomies that provide the content for clinical reasoning.

KEY CONCEPTS

1. The OPT model is a concurrent, iterative thinking model of clinical reasoning that emphasizes reflective self-monitoring as well as framing the context, meaning, and content of clinical reasoning associated with a client story.
2. Client stories provide the backdrop or frame for clinical reasoning.
3. Frames are mental models that influence and guide perception and behavior. Frames determine how we organize and structure our thinking.
4. Critical thinking involves interpretation, analysis, inference, explanation, evaluation, and self-regulation.
5. Reflective clinical reasoning using the OPT model involves the use and application of clinical vocabulary, cue logic, framing, decision making, testing, and judgment.
6. Many thinking strategies support reflective clinical reasoning and critical thinking. Some thinking strategies include drilling, schema search, self-talk, hypothesizing, prototype identification, comparative analysis, reflective verbalization, reframing, if–then thinking, and reflection checks.
7. Integrating critical thinking, reflective reasoning, and the conscious use of thinking strategies supports the use of the OPT model.

STUDY QUESTIONS AND ACTIVITIES

1. Explain why the terms "critical," "creative," and "reflective" thinking are included in the definition of clinical reasoning.

2. Explain in your own words what is meant by the term "concurrent" thinking. Can you think of a metaphor, image, or example of concurrent thinking?

3. Explain differences between problems and outcomes and how the two are related.

4. Explain your cue logic preferences. Are you more comfortable using concepts and general principles to guide your actions, or do you enjoy putting pieces of data together to develop a conclusion? Are you better at deduction or induction?

5. An essential part of the OPT model is testing. How do you create tests or side-by-side comparisons in your own life? What sort of tests do you create to judge the effect of your actions and behaviors? What are the differences between creating a test and making a judgment about the evidence derived from a test? Can you think of an example from your own life?

REFERENCES

Dilts, D. B., Epstein, T., & Dilts, D. W. (1991). *Tools for dreamers: Strategies for creativity and the structure of innovation.* Cupertino, CA: Meta Publications.

Facione, N. C., & Facione, P. A. (1996). Externalizing the critical thinking in knowledge development and clinical judgment. *Nursing Outlook, 44*(3), 129–136.

Fairhurst, G., & Sarr, R. (1996). *The art of framing.* San Francisco, CA: Jossey-Bass.

Fowler, L. (1994). *Clinical reasoning of home health nurses: A verbal protocol analysis.* Unpublished doctoral dissertation, University of South Carolina, College of Nursing Columbia, SC.

Fowler, L., & Herman, J. A. (June, 1995). Reflective verbalization. Paper presented at Fifth Annual Institute on Critical Thinking. Durham, University of New Hampshire.

Giurgevich, P. (1996). Perspectives on dichotomous thinking. *Nurse Education, 21*(4), 41–44.

Herman, J., Pesut, D., & Conard, L. (1994). Using metacognitive skills: The quality audit tool. *Nursing Diagnosis, 5*(2), 56–64.

Lunney, M. (1989). Self-monitoring of accuracy using an integrated model of the diagnostic process. *Journal of Advanced Medical-Surgical Nursing, 1*(3), 43–52.

Miller, G., Galanter, E., & Pribram, K. (1960). *Plans and the structure of behavior.* New York: Holt, Rinehart & Winston.

North American Nursing Diagnosis Association. (1996). *Nursing diagnoses: Definitions and classifications.* Philadelphia: North American Nursing Diagnosis Association.

Pesut, D., Herman, J. A., & Fowler, L. (1996). Toward a revolution in thinking: The OPT model of clinical reasoning. In J. McCloskey & H. Grace (Eds.), *Current issues in nursing* (5th ed., pp. 88–92). St. Louis, MO: Mosby.

Pesut, D. (1989). Aim versus blame: Using an outcome specification model. *Journal of Psychosocial Nursing and Mental Health Services, 27*(5), 26–30.

Senge, P. (1990). *The fifth discipline.* New York: Doubleday.

Walker, L. O., & Avant, K. C. (1995). *Strategies for theory construction in nursing.* Norwalk, CT: Appleton & Lange.

CHAPTER 4

Knowledge Work and Clinical Reasoning: Using Organized Knowledge in Nursing Practice

COMPETENCIES

After completing this chapter, the reader should be able to:

1. Explain why knowledge classification systems are important for organized nursing knowledge.

2. Describe types and levels of classification systems and their consequences for nursing practice.

3. Explain why knowledge work and the clinical vocabulary contained in classification systems are important for clinical reasoning.

4. Describe general features of the following classification systems: NANDA, NIC, NOC, Gordon's functional health patterns, the Omaha Classification System, and the *DSM-IV* system.

5. Explain how nursing knowledge and other classification systems support the science and art of nursing practice.

INTRODUCTION

In this chapter we review the history of classification system development in nursing. Levels of nursing practice data are described. Different levels of nursing practice data are used in making decisions, allocating resources, and contributing to the development of professional nursing practice. Some of the more prominent nursing knowledge classification systems are described. In addition, we describe the *Diagnostic Statistical Manual of Mental Disorders-IV*. Nurses who work in psychiatric mental health settings find this knowledge classification system useful. Finally, we note that the knowledge work and clinical vocabulary that is evolving in these classification systems is the foundation for clinical reasoning. Clinical reasoning presupposes knowledge work.

KNOWLEDGE CLASSIFICATION SYSTEMS IN HEALTH CARE

There are many classification systems used in the health professions. Classification systems organize and store knowledge, systematically grouping ideas into categories based on shared characteristics or traits. The knowledge stored in these systems is useful for clinical reasoning, practice, and research purposes. There are many ways to categorize client problems. Over the years, there have been a number of classification systems used in nursing. Thinking about body systems is a way to classify and store knowledge about anatomy and physiology. This physiological classification system is the foundation for understanding, describing, and explaining many of the physiological problems or diseases that clients experience.

Disease conditions are classified in the *International Classification of Disease (ICD)* published by the World Health Organization (WHO). The *ICD* is a worldwide statistical disease classification system for all medical conditions, including mental disorders (WHO, 1992). The *Diagnostic and Statistical Manual (DSM)* of the American Psychiatric Association is a classification system with which most mental health nurses are familiar. Current procedural terminology (CPT) codes are organized to define and specify treatments used in patient care. These systems standardize and provide structure for knowledge, thus making it available for use, analysis, description, and evaluation.

NURSING KNOWLEDGE CLASSIFICATION SYSTEMS

Nursing-specific knowledge has developed over the past few years and is stored in a variety of classification systems (McCloskey et al., 1990). Initial classification work evolved from the experiences of practicing nurses (Gebbie & Lavin, 1975). Goals were to develop a standard language for nursing (Lang, 1986). Great strides have been made in organizing nursing knowledge over the past three decades. Specifically, the work of NANDA (1994), NIC (McCloskey & Bulechek, 1996), and NOC (Johnson & Maas, 1997) have made major contributions to the systematic development and classification of nursing knowledge.

Each system has a different purpose and uses specific criteria for classification and evaluation of items in the taxonomy. There are a number of ways to classify terms.

The challenge is to select categories that are useful (Fleishman & Quaintane, 1984). Each system uses various techniques to ensure the reliability and validity of the content. Each system contributes to informed practice for the users. Mastering the knowledge organized in these classification systems is the knowledge work nurses need to do in order to reason about nursing.

Why have a classification system? Mills (1991) argues that taxonomies provide language systems to identify relationships among essential elements and core nursing content. Such a systematic language system describes the culture of nursing. Taxonomies structure thinking and decision making as well as facilitate memory and communication and promote consistency of care. Classification systems provide a means for linkages with other classification systems. As Kerr et al. (1991) observe, the purposes of a taxonomy are to understand one's world, communicate with others, provide information in a systematic manner, and identify gaps and relationships within knowledge. As our knowledge grows, taxonomies evolve and change.

The ANA Steering Committee on Classifications of Nursing Practice Phenomena was organized to

1. support diversity in the development and testing of classification systems to describe nursing phenomena until stable systems evolve
2. collaborate with multiple inter- and intradisciplinary groups in identifying and developing classification systems for health care, as well as monitoring and studying the interrelationships of these systems to nursing classification systems
3. promote or facilitate the classification of human responses that nurses diagnose and treat and for which they assume accountability
4. ensure that classification systems developed or used by the nursing profession are adaptable to the various client/health care delivery situations in hospitals, nursing homes, and primary care facilities
5. promote consistent application of classification schemes that are selected, whether used for reimbursement, peer review, standards development, structuring practice, certification, or other purposes

Classification systems and integrated information systems are the building blocks for transforming data into nursing knowledge (Henry & Costantino, 1997).

An effective health care provider is a knowledge worker. Such a person understands how the different classification systems are developed, used, and relate to each other. In addition, there are elements of nursing care information that are used to establish databases that are important to the continued development of the nursing profession.

Following is a brief discussion of some of the nursing classification systems that are important for you to know in order to practice the art and science of clinical reasoning. But first we challenge you to consider how classification can reveal logic and meaning among a set of elements.

STOP AND THINK

What do the following items have in common? An orange, a yellow Post-it note, Brussel sprouts, red brick, red marble, a rusty Brillo pad, an orange Lifesaver, and salmon fillets?

At first you would not think that these items had anything in common. But on second thought, these items do have characteristics in common. As you begin to compare and contrast these items, you discover common characteristics. For example, what if you used color to classify and organize the items? Another possibility is to think about the shape of the items. How do your classifications change when you use shape instead of color to organize them? A third possibility is to cluster the items into groups by texture. How do your groups change when you use texture instead of color to classify the items? The items take on different meanings when different criteria are used. If you use color as the organizer, you likely clustered together the orange, rusty Brillo pad, and orange Lifesaver. All these items are orange. Red brick, red marble, and salmon fillets are red. Leftover items using color as the organizing system are the yellow Post-it note and the green Brussel sprouts.

Using shape as a way to organize the items, it is likely you grouped the orange, Brussels sprouts, red marble, and Lifesaver together because they are all round. The remaining items are square or rectangular: Post-it note, red brick, rusty Brillo pad, and salmon fillets. Using shape, you were able to classify all the items. It is possible that you may disagree with the placement of Brillo pad in the square category if you use Brillo pads that are round. In addition, the size and shape of salmon fillets vary. These differences of opinion are common in all classification systems.

Think about the items in regard to the criteria of texture. How would you classify them given smooth and rough as the criteria? In terms of those things that are smooth, you would likely group Post-it note, red marble, Lifesaver, and salmon fillet. The rough items are the orange, Brussel sprouts, red brick, and rusty Brillo pad. Now step back and look at these groups. The three classification systems you used are very different, yet each enabled classification of the items. The criteria that one uses provides the meaning for the grouping. Remember, classification systems are a way of combining logic with meaning. So classification systems support the blending of art and science.

KNOWLEDGE WORK: LOGIC AND MEANING, ART AND SCIENCE

In Chapter 1, we quoted Einstein: "If what is seen and experienced is portrayed in the language of logic, we are engaged in science. If it is communicated through forms whose connections are not accessible to the conscious mind, but are recognized intuitively as meaningful, then we are engaged in art." Classification systems contribute to science using the language of logic and contribute to art through the establishment of patterns that have meaning.

As you think about classification systems, it is important to hold in your mind the following questions:

1. What is the purpose of this classification system?
2. What criteria were used when classifying items? (Criteria used to classify the content help define the meaning of the terms.)
3. How reliable are the classifications? (In order to reliably classify content, you must have specific criteria for membership in a certain category.)
4. Is the classification system adequate? (How, specifically is the system evaluated in terms of validity? Internal validity exists when the classification criteria can be used by anyone and the same grouping will occur.)
5. Does the classification system make sense to the informed user?

LEVELS OF NURSING PRACTICE DATA

Organizing nursing knowledge for purposes of practice, education, and research is a professional responsibility. However, there are many different levels at which this knowledge can be organized. Figure 4-1 illustrates these levels.

A useful classification system has a specific purpose as well as well-defined criteria for inclusion of items in categories that consistently and reliably assign items to categories; it also makes sense to informed users. When classification systems meet these criteria, they provide the clinical vocabulary for clinical reasoning and assist the nurse in naming client problems, communicating with peers concerning the client, and communicating with other disciplines concerning the nature of nursing's contribution to care. Clinical testing and evaluation of classification systems for practice is an ongoing professional responsibility.

NIC has developed this model to illustrate three levels of nursing practice data:

- the individual level,
- the unit/organization level,
- the network/state/country level (NIC 1997).

For the purposes of most students and clinicians the individual level is the most important for clinical reasoning. Knowledge in these systems contributes to clinical decision making and documentation of care delivered. Managers and administrators are most interested in the organization- and unit-level data. Administrators and researchers are most interested in the network-, state-, and country-level data. All nurses need to be informed about these levels of practice data because these data taken together help describe and define nursing's contribution to the health care enterprise.

NURSING PRACTICE DATA: THREE LEVELS

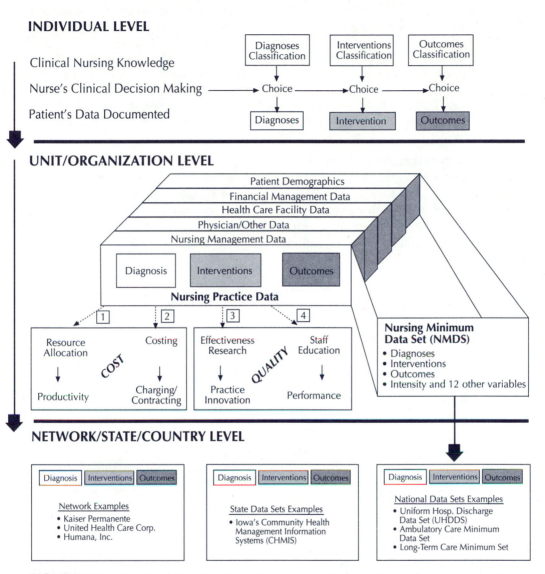

FIGURE 4-1 Levels of Practice Data. Reprinted with Permission from *Image, 29* (3), 1997 228 by the Iowa Nursing Interventions Classification Project. © Iowa Intervention Project, 1997.

Individual Level

The level of immediate interest to most practicing nurses is the individual level. At this level, practice data are organized so that they are relevant and useful in explaining client problems, nursing interventions, outcomes, and clinical choices and decisions that nurses make. Information about the client and the context is explained through the use of clinical knowledge that has been standardized in the form of classification systems or taxonomies. If this information is collected and used according to a standardized system, it can be aggregated and used in a broader context at the unit or organizational level. Developments at this level are expanding as groups and organizations continue to focus on development of nursing diagnoses, interventions, and outcomes.

Unit/Organization Level

At the unit or organizational level, data about individual clients are combined into one system that can be linked to other information systems such as the medical care information system. At this level, analyses about common kinds of treatment can be performed according to four possible parameters: resources, costs, effectiveness, and education. Using data for resource allocation results in measures of productivity. Data related to costs provide information about charging and contracting. Data to support effectiveness research have consequences for practice innovations. Data about staff performance can be used for evaluation and planning. Each institution defines and specifies the type of information most useful for documenting patterns and trends for nursing service in the organization. If you have aspirations to become a nurse-manager these data will be important. What do you think are essential pieces of nursing information? A group of nurse researchers believes a nursing minimum data set is a good place to start. The NMDS is a set of variables with uniform definitions and categories concerning the specific dimensions of nursing which meet the information needs of multiple data users in the macro health care system (Werley & Ryan, 1993). The purpose of the NMDS is to standardize information associated with nursing care that patients receive in a variety of service settings. There are three elements in the data set: nursing care data, client data, and service data.

- Nursing care data elements consist of
  1. nursing diagnosis
  2. nursing intervention
  3. nursing outcome
  4. intensity of nursing care
- Client data elements consist of
  1. personal identification
  2. data of birth, sex, ethnicity, and residence
- Service data elements include
  1. unique facility or service agency number
  2. unique health record of client

3. unique number of principal registered nurse providers
4. episode admission or encounter date
5. discharge date
6. disposition of client
7. expected payer

Network/State/Country Level

The network/state/country level represents the broadest scope of data about nursing activities. At this level, the Nursing Minimum Data Set (NMDS) is used to contribution to the data management needs of many systems.

Benefits of this kind of data set include uniform collection of data that can be compared across a variety of parameters, identification of trends related to client problems and nursing care provided, and reliable data for quality assurance evaluation and costing of nursing service. In addition, such a database promotes comparative research on nursing care, including research on nursing diagnoses, interventions, outcomes, and other clinical nursing research-based questions. Development of the NMDS is a goal toward which many efforts are being channeled. Consequences of this development include a data bank to research projects about nursing care organized at the network, state, country level.

Classification systems provide the content knowledge and clinical vocabulary that is used in clinical reasoning. In the rest of this chapter we introduce classification systems important for clinical reasoning in nursing practice. Realize that your concern at this point in time is at the individual level of practice-relevant data. It is at this level you make choices and decisions about the kind of client problems you identify, the nursing diagnoses you make, the outcomes you establish, and the interventions you choose. In the following chapters, we show how the classification systems are useful.

STOP AND THINK

1. **What would happen if there were no such things as classification systems?**
2. **Why do you think three levels of nursing data are important?**
3. **If you are in a clinical setting now, find out what kinds of individual- or unit-level data are used in the organization.**
4. **Does the data you record on client charts in your clinical setting feed into a larger database or a managed care or health maintenance organization?**
5. **Do you think you would enjoy working on the development of classification systems for nursing knowledge? If so, why? If not, why not?**

NANDA

One of the first nurse-initiated classification systems began in 1973. A group of nurses met in St. Louis, Missouri, and organized the first national conference for the classification of nursing diagnoses. For over twenty years, nurses have been working on developing category labels and diagnoses that reflect patient problems in clinical practice. The first way the diagnoses were categorized was alphabetical. This became cumbersome as new diagnoses were added. Over time, nursing theorists began to look at patterns of diagnoses and in 1984 patterns of unitary man were proposed as an organizing conceptual framework for the diagnostic classification system (Roy, 1984). The patterns are exchanging, communicating, relating, valuing, choosing, moving, perceiving, knowing, and feeling. These patterns represent human responses. Given the 1980 definition of nursing in the ANA social policy statement, human response patterns were introduced to replace the less familiar patterns of unitary man (NANDA, 1994). Following is a brief description of each of the human response patterns and examples of specific nursing diagnoses that fall within that pattern.

BOX 4-1   NANDA Human Response Patterns

Exchanging—mutual giving and receiving
Communicating—sending message
Relating—establishing bonds
Valuing—assigning relative worth
Choosing—selecting alternatives
Moving—activity
Perceiving—reception of information
Knowing—meaning associated with information
Feeling—subjective awareness of information

Source: Kim, M. J., McFarlane, A., & McLane, A. (Eds.). (1984). *Classification of nursing diagnoses: Proceedings of the fifth national conference.* St. Louis, MO: Mosby, p. 29. Reprinted with permission from the North American Diagnosis Association (NANDA) and Nursecom, Inc.

Exchanging is the human response pattern involving mutual giving and receiving. Specific nursing diagnoses under this category include tissue perfusion, impaired gas exchange, ineffective airway clearance, and alteration in nutrition. Communicating is a human response pattern that involves sending messages. An example of a nursing diagnosis under this category is impaired communication. Relating is a human response pattern that involves establishing bonds. Specific examples of diagnoses under this category include social isolation, altered family process, and caregiver role strain. Valuing is a human response pattern that involves the assigning of relative worth or value. An example of a nursing diagnosis within this pattern is spiritual distress. Choosing as a human response pattern involves the selection of alternatives. Examples are ineffective individual coping and ineffective management of therapeutic regimen. Moving involves activity. Nursing diagnoses under this category include such things as impaired physical mobility, activity intolerance, and fatigue. Perceiving as a human response pattern involves the reception of information. Nursing diagnoses in this category include alterations in self-concept and body image as well as a variety of sensory-perceptual alterations. Knowing as a human response pattern involves the meaning associated with information. Examples of diagnoses include knowledge deficit and altered thought processes. The final category of human responses is feeling. Feeling as a human response pattern involves the subjective awareness of information. Examples of diagnoses in this category include such things as pain, grieving, anxiety, and fear (Doenges & Moorhouse, 1996; NANDA, 1994).

The purpose of NANDA is to provide a means to develop, organize, and test nursing diagnoses that are within the independent domain of nursing practice. Criteria are set forth in the procedures to develop and introduce diagnoses to the NANDA community. Reliability of NANDA diagnoses are supported by research literature, validation studies, and periodic refinement of labels and definitions. Labels and categories are tested in order to determine their adequacy. Diagnoses are accepted for clinical testing. As a result of use, diagnoses are tested and refined over time.

NIC

"Classifying nursing treatments is essential for the articulation and advancement of the knowledge base of nursing. Nurses have been doing and documenting care for decades, but in no uniform way. NIC provides a common language to communicate among ourselves and others the important work of nursing" (McCloskey & Bulechek, 1996, p. 41). There are at least six other reasons for a classification system of nursing interventions:

1. to standardize the nomenclature about nursing treatments
2. to expand nursing knowledge about the links among diagnoses, treatments, and outcomes
3. to facilitate the development of nursing information systems
4. to facilitate teaching of decision making to nursing students
5. to determine the cost of services provided by nurses
6. to assist in planning for resources needed in nursing practice settings (McCloskey et al., 1990)

NIC is the first comprehensive standardized classification of treatments that nurses perform. For a discussion of the process and procedures used to create NIC, refer to the work of McCloskey and Bulechek (1996).

Domains

NIC is organized in a three-level taxonomy that includes domains, classes, and interventions. The six domains are the most abstract level of the taxonomy. Domain 1, Physiological: Basic, involves nursing care that supports basic physiological functioning. Examples of classes in this domain include issues related to activity and exercise management, elimination management, immobility management, nutrition support, physical comfort promotion, and self-care facilitation. Specific interventions in these classes are exercise therapy, catheterization, positioning, tube feeding, pain management, and bathing.

Domain 2, Physiological: Complex, involves care that supports complex physiological homeostatic regulation. Examples of classes in this domain include electrolyte and acid base management, drug management, neurological management, peri-operative care, respiratory management, skin and wound management, thermoregulation, and tissue perfusion management. Specific interventions in these classes are hypoglycemia management, analgesic administration, seizure management, postanesthesia care, airway suctioning, incision site care, hypothermia treatment, and fluid monitoring.

Domain 3, Behavioral, involves care that supports psychosocial functioning and facilitates lifestyle changes. Examples of classes in this domain include behavior therapy, cognitive therapy, communication enhancement, coping assistance, patient education, and psychological comfort promotion. Specific interventions in theses classes are assertiveness training, reminiscence therapy, active listening, anticipatory guidance and counseling, teaching, and relaxation therapy.

Domain 4, Safety, involves care that supports protection against harm. There are only two classes in this domain: crisis management and risk management. An example of crisis management intervention is code management. An example of a risk management intervention is seizure management.

Domain 5, Family, involves care that supports the family unit. Classes in this domain are childbearing care and life span care. Life span care involves interventions to facilitate family unit functioning and promote the health and welfare of family members throughout the life span. Specific interventions associated with these two classes include childbirth preparation and caregiver support.

The sixth and final domain, Health System, is care that supports the effective use of the health care system. Classes in this domain are health system mediation, health system management, and information management. Interventions associated with each of these classes include patient rights protection, staff supervision and peer review, and documentation (McCloskey & Bulechek, 1996).

A recent study compared nursing intervention classification and CPT codes for categorizing nursing activities. Results provided evidence that the NIC classification system was superior to the CPT system (Henry, Holzemer, Randell, Hsieh, & Miller, 1997).

NOC

A research team at the University of Iowa is doing important work regarding nursing-sensitive patient outcomes classification. Nursing-sensitive patient outcomes are variable patient or family states, behaviors, or perceptions responsive to nursing interventions and conceptualized at middle levels of abstraction (Johnson & Maas, 1997). Nursing outcomes are one element needed to complete the Nursing Minimum Data Set (NMDS).

The purpose of the Iowa NOC project is to identify, label, validate, and classify patient-sensitive outcomes and indicators; evaluate the validity and usefulness of the outcomes classification through clinical field testing; and define and test measurement procedures for the outcomes and indicators. The researchers developed outcomes as variable concepts so client states in response to nursing interventions could be documented over time and across contexts.

Each outcome is associated with a group of indicators used to determine the outcome. For example, fluid balance as an outcome is defined as balance of water in the intracellular and extracellular components of the body. Thinking of this on a continuum, five degrees of fluid balance are scaled. The range includes (1) extremely compromised, (2) substantially compromised, (3) compromised, (4) moderately compromised, (5) not compromised. Use of a scaling method provides quantifiable information about outcome achievement.

Indicators that fall under the fluid balance outcome definition include: mean arterial and central venous pressure, pulmonary wedge pressure, 24-hour intake and output balance, body weight, presence or absence of sunken eyes, thirst, edema, or neck vein distention.

NOC work is on the cutting edge and contributes a very important piece to the knowledge work that is needed in nursing. Combing the work of NANDA, NIC, and NOC is important clinical scholarship for the next century.

NANDA diagnoses, NIC interventions, and NOC outcome classifications provide the clinical vocabulary for clinical reasoning in nursing. The OPT model provides the structure and some of the thinking strategies for integrating these classification systems in the service of care. For more information about NOC, go to the Internet http://www.nursing.uiowa.edu/

THE OMAHA CLASSIFICATION SYSTEM

The Omaha classification system was developed by integrating thoughts and ideas from nursing theorists, researchers, community health nursing educators, and staff and supervisory nurses of the Visiting Nurses Association of Omaha (Martin & Scheet, 1992). The model is an approach to community health nursing. The three parts of the classification scheme are: problem classification , intervention scheme, and problem rating scale for outcomes (Martin & Scheet, 1992).

In the Omaha system, four categories organize community health nursing practice. The categories or domains represent the first level of the problem classification scheme. These are environmental, psychosocial, physiological, and health-related behaviors. Within each defined domain, there are specified problems. Each problem can be placed on a continuum that ranges from deficit to health promotion. The second modifier identifies the focus of the problem as an individual or a family. Finally, associated signs and symptoms provide diagnostic clues to problem identification.

BOX 4-2   Omaha Classification System Domains and Interventions.

Domains
    Environmental
        Material resources
        Physical surroundings
    Psychosocial
        Patterns of behavior
        Communication
        Relationships
        Development
    Physiological
        Process that maintain life
    Health-Related Behavior
        Behaviors that maintain or promote wellness, recovery, rehabilitation
Interventions
    Health Teaching
        Giving information, responsibility for self-care
    Guidance and Counseling
        Anticipating client problems, coping
    Treatment and Procedures
        Prevention, identification, and alleviation of signs and symptoms
    Case Management and Surveillance
        Coordination, advocacy, referral

Reprinted with permission from ANA.

The environmental domain considers material resources and the physical surroundings of the client's home, neighborhood, and community. Examples of problems in this domain are income, sanitation, residence, and neighborhood workplace safety. For example, signs and symptoms associated with identification of neighborhood safety problems include high crime rate, unsafe play areas, and physical hazards. The problem would be a deficit in neighborhood safety.

The psychosocial domain involves patterns of behavior, communication, relationships, and development. Twelve problems in this area are: communication with community resources, social contact, role change, interpersonal relationships, spiritual distress, grief, emotional stability, human sexuality, caretaking/parenting, neglected child/adult, abused child/adult, growth and development, and other. For example, signs and symptoms that enable one to identify communication with community resources include language barriers, dissatisfaction with services, or unfamiliarity with procedures for obtaining services. The problem would be impairment regarding communication with community resources.

The physiological domain involves processes that maintain life. Problems in this domain are usually associated with the individual rather than the family. There are fifteen problems, which focus on physical health status. Specific problems include hearing, vision, speech and language, dentition, cognition, pain, consciousness, integument, neuromusculoskeletal function, respiration, circulation, digestion/hydration, bowel function, genitourinary, antepartum/postpartum, and other. For example, limited range of motion and decreased muscle strength are indicative of impaired neuromusculoskeletal function.

The health-related behaviors domain involves behaviors that maintain or promote wellness, recovery, or rehabilitation. Specific problems in this domain include nutrition, sleep and rest patterns, physical activity, personal hygiene, substance use, family planning, health care supervision, prescribed medication regimen, technical procedure, and other. A sedentary lifestyle would be a sign indicative of impairment with physical activity.

The intervention scheme is a framework of nursing actions for use with nursing diagnoses. There are four categories of nursing interventions: health teaching, guidance and counseling, treatment and procedures, case management and surveillance. Health teaching, guidance, and counseling involve such activities as giving information, anticipating client problems, responsibility for self-care, and coping. Treatments and procedures are actions directed toward prevention, identification, and alleviation of signs and symptoms. Case management includes nursing activities of coordination, advocacy, and referral. Surveillance includes detection, measurement, critical analysis, and monitoring to indicate client status in relation to a given client condition.

The purpose of the Omaha system was to provide community health nurses with a systematic way to classify and code problems and interventions relevant to community and home health care nursing practice. Criteria were developed based on problems, interventions, and a problem rating scale for outcomes. The system is receiving increased attention in terms of its reliability, adaptability, and cohesiveness to practitioners in the field (Martin, Leak, & Aden, 1992).

GORDON'S FUNCTIONAL HEALTH PATTERNS

Concurrent with the development of the NANDA classification system, Marjorie Gordon developed a format for client assessment that organized data for the purposes of identifying nursing diagnoses (Gordon, 1994). Gordon's functional health patterns can also be considered a classification system. She identified 11 patterns of health and illness to describe client responses over time. The health perception/health management pattern describes the client's perceived pattern of health and well-being and how health is managed. Diagnoses in this category are potential for infection, health management deficit, and altered health maintenance.

BOX 4-3   Typology of Gordon's Eleven Functional Health Patterns

- Health perception/health management pattern—client's perceived pattern of health and well-being and how health is managed
- Nutritional/metabolic pattern—pattern of food and fluid consumption relative to metabolic need and pattern indicators of local nutrient supply
- Elimination pattern—patterns of excretory function (bowel, bladder, and skin)
- Activity/exercise pattern—pattern of exercise, activity, leisure, and recreation
- Sleep/rest pattern—patterns of sleep, rest, and relaxation
- Cognitive/perceptual pattern—sensory-perceptual and cognitive pattern
- Self-perception/self-concept pattern—self-concept pattern and perceptions of self (e.g., body comfort, body image, feeling state)
- Role/relationship pattern—pattern of role-engagements and relationships
- Sexuality/reproductive pattern—client's patterns of satisfaction and dissatisfaction with sexuality pattern; describes reproductive patterns
- Coping/stress tolerance pattern—general coping pattern and effectiveness of the pattern in terms of stress tolerance
- Value/belief pattern—pattern of values, beliefs (including spiritual), or goals that guide choices or decisions

Reprinted with permission from Gordon, M. (1994). *Nursing diagnosis: Process and application*. St. Louis, MO: Mosby. From *Manual of Nursing Diagnosis*, by M. Gordon, 1997, St. Louis, MO: Mosby-Yearbook, Inc.

The nutritional/metabolic pattern describes the client's pattern of fluid and food consumption. This category includes the condition of skin, hair, nails, and mucus membranes and teeth as well as measurements of body temperature and weight. Diagnoses in this category include fluid volume deficit, potential skin breakdown, and impaired swallowing. The elimination pattern describes patterns of excretory elimination, including bowel, bladder, and skin. Specific diagnoses in this category are constipation, diarrhea, and functional incontinence. The activity/exercise pattern includes activities of daily living, including expenditure of energy. Also included are the type and quantity of exercise and any deficit that would impair activity. Examples of diagnoses in this category are self-care deficit, activity intolerance, and diversional activity deficit.

The sleep/rest pattern describes perceptions and patterns of the quality and quantity of rest/relaxation periods over a 24-hour period. An example of diagnoses in this category is sleep pattern disturbance. The cognitive/perceptual pattern describes the adequacy of sensory modes such as vision, hearing, taste, touch, or smell and any supports needed to deal with deficits. This category also includes pain perception, language, memory, judgment, and decision-making issues. Examples in this category are pain, decisional conflict, and confusion. The self-perception/self-concept pattern includes attitudes and perceptions about self, image, identity, worth, and emotions. Diagnoses in this category include anxiety, powerlessness, and body image disturbance. The role/relationship pattern includes perception of adequacy of and satisfaction with role functioning. Examples of nursing diagnoses in this category are impaired communication, altered family process, and grieving.

The sexuality/reproductive pattern describes human functioning and satisfaction with sexuality and sexual relationships. Conditions associated with female reproductive states are also included. Diagnoses in this category include sexual dysfunction and altered patterns of sexuality. The coping/stress tolerance pattern includes the individual's ability to manage, control, and handle stress. Examples of diagnoses under this category include ineffective individual coping, caregiver role strain, and impaired adjustment. The final category is the value/belief pattern, which describes the individual's perception of what is important in life, health values, and any expectations that are health-related. Spiritual beliefs are included in this category. Nursing diagnoses in this category are spiritual distress and potential for enhanced spiritual well-being.

DSM-IV

The previous classification systems evolved from the nursing profession's desire to identify, define, and classify those human responses unique to nursing practice. Mental health problems have their own unique classification history and system (Sapp, 1996a; 1996b).

Psychiatric mental health nurses developed a task force to examine phenomena of concern to mental health nurses. This effort led to beginning work on a classification system of human responses of interest to psychiatric mental health nurses (O'Toole & Loomis, 1989; Lego, 1996). The work begun by this task force has been assumed by NANDA.

The *DSM* evolved over the years. This system uses a multi-axial approach to clinical diagnosis. Clients often have more than one problem or exhibit different degrees of stress and coping responses in response to stressors. The *DSM-IV* takes the multifocal aspects of client problems and organizes them around five axes. Diagnostic conclusions based on analysis and assessment of the interaction among the five axes gives the clinician a greater understanding of the client (Pies, 1994). This multi-axial approach illustrates how conditions interact and influence other conditions. (Refer to Table 4-1.)

Axes I and II comprise all the mental disorders and other conditions that are the focus of attention. For example, an Axis I diagnosis might be major depression. An Axis II diagnosis might be antisocial personality. Axis III is a way to document and record the patient's general medical condition from the *ICD*. Examples include heart disease, hypertension, or diabetes. Axis IV provides categories of psychosocial and environmental problems such as occupational, educational, or economic problems. Axis V provides an assessment scale that can be used to judge (on a 0–100 point scale) a client's global assessment or overall function. Given recent changes in health care, there has been an emphasis on primary care and prevention. To this end a

TABLE 4-1 DSM-IV Axis I–IV Disorders

AXIS I
Clinical Disorders
Other Conditions That May Be a
  Focus of Clinical Attention
Disorders Usually First
  Diagnosed in Infancy, Child-
  hood, or Adolescence
(Excluding Mental Retardation,
  which is diagnosed on Axis II)
Delirium, Dementia, and
  Amnestic and Other Cognitive
  Disorders
Mental Disorders Due to a
  General Medical Condition
Substance-Related Disorders
Schizophrenia and Other
  Psychotic Disorders
Mood Disorders
Anxiety Disorders
Somatoform Disorders
Factitious Disorders
Dissociative Disorders
Sexual and Gender Identity
  Disorders
Eating Disorders
Sleep Disorders
Impulse-Control Disorders Not
  Elsewhere Classified
Adjustment Disorders
Other Conditions That May Be a
  Focus of Clinical Attention

AXIS II
Personality Disorders
Mental Retardation
Paranoid Personality Disorder
Dependent Personality Disorder
Schizoid Personality Disorder
Obsessive-Compulsive
  Personality Disorder
Schizotypal Personality Disorder
Personality Disorder Not
  Otherwise Specified
Antisocial Personality Disorder
Borderline Personality Disorder
Histrionic Personality Disorder
Narcissistic Personality Disorder
Mental Retardation
Avoidant Personality Disorder

AXIS III
General Medical Conditions (with
  ICD-9-CM codes)
Infectious and Parasitic Diseases
  (001-139)
Neoplasms (140-239)
Endocrine, Nutritional, and

AXIS IV
Psychosocial and Environmental
  Problems
Problems with Primary Support
  Group
Problems Related to the Social
  Environment

continued

TABLE 4-1 *(continued)*

(AXIS III *continued*)
Metabolic Diseases and Immunity Disorders (240-279)
Diseases of the Blood and Blood-Forming Organs (280-289)
Diseases of the Nervous System and Sense Organs (320-389)
Diseases of the Circulatory System (390-459)
Diseases of the Respiratory System (460-519)
Diseases of the Digestive System (520-579)
Diseases of the Genitourinary System (580-629)
Complications of Pregnancy, Childbirth, and the Puerperium (630-676)
Diseases of the Skin and Subcutaneous Tissue (680-709)
Diseases of the Musculoskeletal System and Connective Tissue (710-739)
Congenital Anomalies (740-759)
Certain Conditions Originating in the Perinatal Period (760-779)
Symptoms, Signs, and Ill-Defined Conditions (780-799)
Injury and Poisoning (800-999)

(AXIS IV *continued*)
Educational Problems
Occupational Problems
Housing Problems
Economic Problems
Problems with Access to Health Care Services
Problems Related to Interaction with the Legal System/Crime
Other Psychosocial and Environmental Problems

Reprinted with permission from the *Diagnostic and Statistical Manual of Mental Disorders, Fourth Edition.* Copyright 1994 American Psychiatric Association.

primary care version of *DSM-IV* has been developed (American Psychiatric Association, 1994).

Wilson and Kneisl (1996) offer the following observations about the usefulness of the *DSM-IV* for nursing. It provides a framework for interdisciplinary communication. It is well tested in the field and has demonstrated reliability and validity. The classification system represents a more progressive, holistic view of mind–body relations.

The *DSM-IV* provides for diagnostic certainty, and incorporates biological, psychological, and social variables. The system considers an individual's adaptive strengths as well as problems, and reflects a descriptive phenomenological perspective rather than any psychiatric theory (Wilson & Kneisl, 1996, p. 147). What the *DSM-IV* does not do is assist one in identifying the nursing knowledge work that is associated with care of persons with mental disorders.

CLASSIFICATION SYSTEMS AND KNOWLEDGE WORK

Each of the knowledge classification systems discussed in this chapter represents the kind of data health care providers must use in their knowledge work. All of this knowledge has relevance for clinical reasoning in nursing. For example, NANDA has approved over 100 nursing diagnoses that are supported for clinical testing. These nursing diagnoses are the patterns of human responses nurses have witnessed in clinical care contexts. NIC has systematically culled the literature and validated over 433 nursing interventions that describe what nurses do and how nurses intervene.

The Omaha classification system uniquely describes the domains and factors of concern to nurses who practice in community health. A possible focus on the environment and community as well as case management and surveillance makes this system appealing to practitioners in community settings.

Gordon's functional health patterns system provides an approach to assessment that revolves around patterns of behavior rather than problem-focused areas. Her 11 functional health patterns approach helps clinicians target deviations and generate hypotheses that can be tested regarding more specific problem-focused areas of patient care.

Finally, mental disorders cut across disciplines. Psychiatrists, psychologists, social workers, and nurses need a working knowledge of the behavior and characteristics of mental disorders. To this end *DSM-IV* provides knowledge as well as a multi-axial way to think about the complexity and interaction among the dimensions of mental disorders, personality, medical condition, stressors, and contexts of a given client situation. Each of these systems was developed with a specific purpose in mind. Each established criteria to ensure reliability, adequacy, and usefulness for clinicians in practice. Each represents a system that stores specific knowledge that is useful to clinicians as they reason about client problems, interventions, and outcomes.

How one uses the knowledge stored in these classifications systems depends on one's practice context, knowledge, beliefs, values, and professional identity. As nursing continues to evolve, classification systems become an important focus of clinical scholarship. Members of the profession have an obligation and responsibility to stay informed, use, and refine the knowledge contained in these systems. The knowledge stored in these systems is the vocabulary of and for clinical reasoning. As you will see in subsequent chapters the OPT model provides a structure that can use knowledge classification systems in an artful way.

SUMMARY

The 1990s have seen tremendous development and change in the creation of nursing knowledge and diagnoses. A series of projects resulted in the development of nursing classification systems such as the NANDA taxonomy, the Omaha classification system for home health, and Gordon's functional health patterns. Through systematic research and peer review, these taxonomies developed labels, defining characteristics, and created structures that organized some of the most fundamental client problems that nurses deal with on a day-to-day basis. Taxonomies have several advantages. Taxonomies give nursing a professional identity. They provide a structure to store knowledge and a common language. Taxonomies define the nature of nursing care. Taxonomies are coded so that it is possible to link payment to services and link nursing to other databases and health care classification systems. Taxonomies provide the content one uses in clinical reasoning. With many problems already identified, the nature of nursing process changed from problem solving to reasoning about relationships among problems, interventions, and outcomes in the context of a client's story.

KEY CONCEPTS

1. The development of classification systems is important in order to standardize language about nursing diagnoses, interventions, and outcomes.
2. When examining a classification system, pay attention to the following issues: purpose, criteria used to create categories, classes, reliability, adaptability, coherence or sense to the user.
3. In addition to classification systems, there are three levels of nursing practice data relevant to nurses: the individual level; the unit or organization level; and the local, state, or national level.
4. NANDA is the professional organization sanctioned by the ANA to develop nursing diagnoses.
5. Gordon's functional health patterns provide a means of assessment based on patterns of behavior.
6. NIC is a recent classification that focuses on nursing intervention in six domains.
7. NOC is a recent classification system that categorizes nurse-sensitive patient outcomes.
8. NANDA diagnoses, NIC interventions, and NOC outcome classifications provide the clinical vocabulary for clinical reasoning in nursing. The OPT model provides the structure and some of the cognitive processes for integrating these classification systems in the service of care.
9. The Omaha classification system was developed to uniquely address the problems, intervention scheme, and nursing actions of home health nurses.
10. *DSM-IV* uses a multi-axial approach to client assessment. While it is helpful

to determine diagnoses, it is not specific in regard to identification of nursing care needs of clients who have mental disorders.

11. Knowing the knowledge contained in these systems makes clinical reasoning easier, more effective, and more efficient. Knowledge stored or classified in these systems is the content for clinical reasoning.

STUDY QUESTIONS AND ACTIVITIES

1. Which of the knowledge classification systems described in this chapter are you most familiar with? Make a list of the advantages and disadvantages of each system described in this chapter.

2. Conduct a literature search on the system you know the least about. Find out what current information exists regarding this system.

3. Conduct a debate on the question of whether *DSM-IV* is a relevant knowledge classification system for nurses.

4. One of the disadvantages of classification systems is that they promote labeling of individuals given certain diagnoses. Discuss with a classmate the pros and cons of "labeling" clients using existing classification system terminology.

5. Interview someone in another discipline and ask if they use knowledge classification systems in their work.

REFERENCES

American Psychiatric Association. (1994). *Diagnostic and statistical manual of mental disorders* (4th ed.). Washington, DC: American Psychiatric Association.

Doenges, M., & Moorhouse, M. (1996). *Nurses pocket guide: Nursing diagnoses with interventions*. Philadelphia, PA: Davis.

Fitzpatrick, J. (1991). Taxonomy II: Definitions and development. In R. Carroll-Johnson (Ed.), *Classification of nursing diagnoses: Proceedings of the ninth conference* (pp. 23–29). Philadelphia, PA: Lippincott.

Fleishman, E. A., & Quaintance, M. K. (1984). *Taxonomies of human performance*. New York: Academic.

Gebbie, K. M., & Lavin, M. A. (1975). *Classification of nursing diagnoses: Proceedings of the first national conference*. St. Louis, MO: Mosby.

Gordon, M. (1994). *Nursing diagnosis: Process and application*. St. Louis, MO: Mosby.

Henry, S., & Constantino, M. (1997). Classification systems and integrated information systems: Building blocks for transforming data into nursing knowledge. In J. McCloskey & H. Grace (Eds.), *Current issues in nursing* (5th ed., pp. 74–87). St. Louis, MO: Mosby.

Henry, S., Holzemer, W., Randell, C., Hsieh, S., & Miller, T. (1997). Comparison of nursing interventions classification and current procedural terminology codes for categorizing nursing activities. *Image: Journal of Nursing Scholarship, 29*(2), 133–138.

Johnson, M., & Maas, M. (Eds.). (1997). *Nursing outcomes classification*. St. Louis, MO: Mosby.

Kerr, M. (1991). Validation of taxonomies. In R. Carroll-Johnson (Ed.), *Classification of nursing diagnoses: Proceedings of the ninth conference* (pp. 6–13). Philadelphia, PA: Lippincott.

Lang, N. (1986). Classification, taxonomy, structure. In M. E. Hurley (Ed.), *Classification of nursing diagnoses: Proceedings of the sixth conference* (pp. 14–22). St. Louis, MO: Mosby.

Lego, S. (1996). Appendix C: Classification of human responses of concern for psychiatric mental health nursing. In S. Lego (Ed.), *Psychiatric nursing: A comprehensive reference* (pp. 607–612). Philadelphia, PA: Lippincott.

Martin, K., Leak, G., & Aden, C. (1992). The Omaha system: A research based model for decision making. *Journal of Nursing Administration, 22*(11), 47–52.

Martin, K., & Scheet, N. J. (1992). *The Omaha system: Applications for community health nursing*. Orlando, FL: Saunders.

McCloskey, J. C., & Bulechek, G. M. (1996). *Nursing intervention classification* (2nd ed.). St. Louis, MO: Mosby.

McCloskey, J. C., Bulechek, G. M., Cohen, M., Craft, M., Crossley, J., Denehy, J., Glick, O., Kruckeberg, T., Maas, M., Prophet, C., & Tripp-Reiner, T. (1990). Classification of nursing interventions. *Journal of Professional Nursing, 6*(3), 151–157.

Mills, W. (1991). Why a classification system? In R. Carroll-Johnson (Ed.), *Classification of nursing diagnoses: Proceedings of the ninth conference* (pp. 3–6). Philadelphia, PA: Lippincott.

North American Nursing Diagnosis Association. (1994). *Nursing diagnoses: Definitions and classification, 1994–1996*. Philadelphia: North American Nursing Diagnosis Association.

Nursing Interventions Classification (NIC) Project Newsletter (1995). *3*(3–4).

O'Toole, A., & Loomis, M. (1989). Revision of the phenomena of concern for psychiatric mental health nursing. *Archives of Psychiatric Nursing, 3*(5), 288–299.

Pies, R. (1994) *Clinical manual of psychiatric diagnosis and treatment*. Washington, DC: American Psychiatric Press.

Roy, C., Sr. (1984). Framework for classification systems development: Progress and issues. In M. Kim, A. McFarlane, & A. McLane (Eds.), *Classification of nursing diagnoses: Proceedings of the fifth national conference* (pp. 26–58). St. Louis, MO: Mosby.

Sapp, J. (1996a). Diagnosis and the *DSM-IV*. In S. Lego (Ed.), *Psychiatric nursing: A comprehensive reference* (pp. 14–26). Philadelphia, PA: Lippincott.

Sapp, J. (1996b). Psychiatric nursing assessment. In S. Lego (Ed.), *Psychiatric nursing: A comprehensive reference* (pp. 3–14). Philadelphia, PA: Lippincott.

Sokal, R. R. (1974). Classification: Purposes, principles, progress, prospects. *Science, 185,* 1114–1123.

Wilson, H., & Kneisl, C. (1996). Psychiatric nursing (5th ed.). Menlo Park, CA: Addision-Wesley.

World Health Organization. (1992). *Manual of the international classification of diseases and related health problems* (10th rev. ed.). Geneva, Switzerland: WHO.

Werley, H., Ryan, P., Zorn, C., & Devine, E. (1994). *Why the nursing minimum data set?* In J. McClosky & H. K. Grace (Eds.), *Current issues in nursing* (4th ed., pp. 113–122). St. Louis, MO: Mosby.

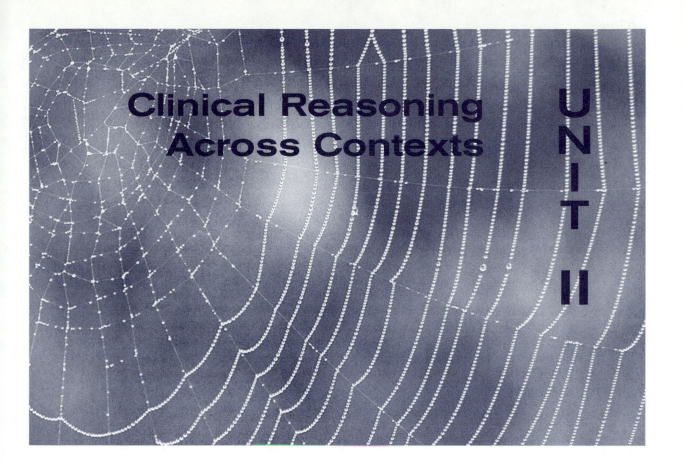

Clinical Reasoning Across Contexts

UNIT II

Unit II consists of six chapters. In Chapter 5, we put the OPT model to use in clinical practice and introduce several tools that support the model's use. We explain the use of a Clinical Reasoning Web, the OPT Model Worksheet, and the Thinking Strategies Worksheet. In Chapter 6, we apply the OPT model to a case story in a primary care context. In Chapter 7, we apply the OPT model to a case story in the acute care context. In Chapter 8, we apply the OPT model to a case story in community health. In Chapter 9, we apply the OPT model to a case story in community mental health. In Chapter 10, we apply the OPT model to a case story in long-term care context. In each story we note the steps one takes as one reflects and reasons about the nursing care needs of clients in different contexts.

Quick Reference Table of Contents for Unit II

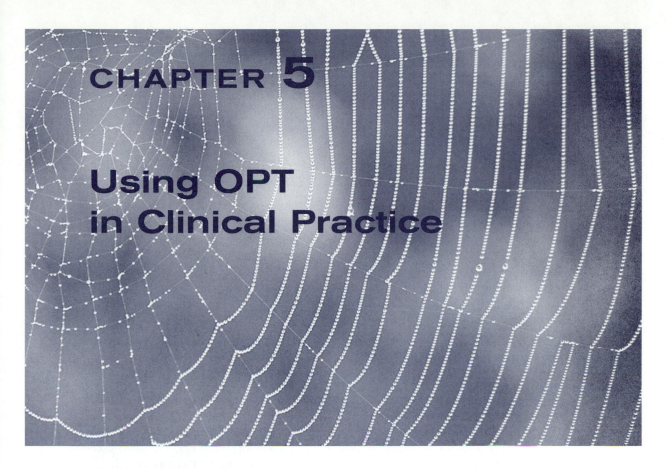

CHAPTER 5

Using OPT in Clinical Practice

COMPETENCIES

After completing this chapter, the reader should be able to:

1. Explain how the OPT model provides a structure for nursing knowledge.
2. Describe the process of spinning and weaving a Clinical Reasoning Web.
3. Explain how to use the OPT model, Clinical Reasoning Web, and Thinking Strategies Worksheet to reason about a specific case study.
4. Use the OPT Model Worksheet, Clinical Reasoning Web, and Thinking Strategies Worksheet to record data on a selected client situation.
5. Define and give an example of each of the thinking strategies that support reflective clinical reasoning.
6. Conduct a reflection check to evaluate the application of critical and creative thinking skills to a selected clinical case study.

INTRODUCTION

In this chapter we show you how to use the OPT model with a clinical case. We discuss the importance of knowing the clinical vocabulary contained in nursing classification systems. We explain how the OPT model provides the organization and structure for clinical reasoning. We introduce you to some strategies, techniques, and worksheets that will assist you in mastering clinical reasoning skills. Finally, as we work through a case study, we challenge you to monitor the critical and creative thinking that supports clinical reasoning.

CLINICAL REASONING: CREATING STRUCTURE FOR YOUR KNOWLEDGE WORK

Reasoning is complex and is subject to variation based on knowledge, skill, and experience. Reasoning involves knowledge and structure. Some, but not all knowledge work necessary for nursing is contained in the knowledge classification systems organized by NANDA, NIC, and NOC. Knowledge classification and development in nursing is an ongoing evolutionary process. As new nursing knowledge is defined, classified, and stored in classification systems it becomes part of the words or clinical vocabulary with which one reasons. The structure of the OPT model accommodates contemporary nursing knowledge development activities in various ways. OPT can be used in education, practice, and research contexts.

KNOWLEDGE WORK AND THE OPT MODEL

One of the challenges of professional nursing practice is keeping abreast of progress in the area of knowledge pertinent to the profession. The classification system one uses provides the content and focus through which you see the world and reason about clients. It is not possible to reason without knowing what knowledge is contained in these classification systems. Reasoning without classification knowledge is like trying to learn a language without knowing the words or the alphabet.

Nursing and other knowledge classification systems provide the clinical vocabulary for clinical reasoning. Become aware of the classification filters you use. You may not even be aware or conscious of them! Many nursing assessment forms use a body systems approach to structure data collection, determine problems, and organize nursing care. Do you organize nursing care around body systems? Is this a nursing or medical approach to care?

Institutions have their own assessment forms or checklists. Use of standardized forms creates a lens through which assessments are made and data are gathered. Such forms organize the knowledge that is deemed necessary by the institution. Such organization directly influences thinking and reasoning. The knowledge classification system one uses is a filter through which situations are defined, analyzed, and evaluated. For example, Gordon's functional health patterns is a useful model for assessments and is a fine way to begin to think about and frame client care needs. If you use NANDA, you will be thinking in terms such as exchanging, communicating, relating, and valuing. A NANDA diagnosis of self-care deficit structures thinking in a specific way.

A *DSM-IV* diagnosis of depression or obsessive compulsive disorder organizes thinking about a client in a different way. *DSM-IV* serves as a useful system for mental disorders. However, not every nurse is familiar with this classification system. Nurses treat more than mental disorders so other classification/knowledge systems are needed to describe, explain, and document the nursing care needs of clients across different contexts.

If you provide care in the context of community or are involved in home health nursing, the Omaha classification system is helpful for organizing thinking and care planning. The Omaha system organizes issues around problems in the areas of physiological processes, psychosocial patterns, environmental issues, and health-related behaviors. Each classification system conceptualizes client needs, issues, and nursing problems in a different way and approaches care in a slightly different way.

STOP AND THINK

1. **Which nursing knowledge classification systems do you like and use the most?**
2. **In your own words, how do you explain the differences among the nursing knowledge classification systems with which you are familiar?**
3. **What are some of the ways you can learn the knowledge and categories in each of the classification systems we have described?**

THE OPT MODEL: A STRUCTURE FOR CLINICAL REASONING

The OPT model accommodates the knowledge classified in the NANDA, NIC, and NOC taxonomies. As knowledge work in nursing grows and develops, we believe our model will be a useful tool that provides a structure that enables one to put the pieces of the many patient care puzzles together. Clinical reasoning tools help nurses reason effectively. Tools help one think systematically about the clients, their stories, and the issues clients share. Clinical reasoning involves many tasks. For example, one needs a way to gather and keep track of data, discern the issues, and make decisions. Reasoning is like drawing a map or planning a trip. If you know where you are and you know where you want to go, there are many ways to get there.

Think of the OPT model as a way to help you identify where you are and where you want to go with your clients. Based on the facts of the situation you have choices to make in order to get to your destination. The first challenge of clinical reasoning is to represent all the issues and needs that clients reveal. The second challenge is to consider how all these issues are related to one another. The third challenge is to find the keystone issue that organizes the focus of your care based on the client's story.

Once the keystone issue is identified, other diagnostic concerns may be resolved through activities surrounding the keystone issue.

We have created three worksheets that help meet the challenges we have set forth. The OPT Model Worksheet provides an organizational framework for the reasoning task. The Clinical Reasoning Web helps determine relationships among issues and reveal what the keystone issue might be. The Thinking Strategies Worksheet helps you reflect and monitor your own use and application of thinking strategies. Together with the OPT model, these learning tools help you master the art and science of clinical reasoning.

OPT Model Worksheet

The OPT Model Worksheet was designed to provide a pictorial representation or map of the structure of the OPT model. Think of it as a guide to help structure your thinking. Box 5-1 lists questions that guide reflective clinical reasoning. Answers to these questions help you complete the information that can be inserted in the spaces in the OPT Model Worksheet shown in Figure 5-1.

BOX 5-1   Questions That Guide the Use of the OPT Model

Client-in-Context

1. What is the client's story?
2. What cues are associated with the client's story?

Cue Logic

1. What taxonomy was used to structure and give meaning to the cues?
2. Which specific cues verify present-state inferences or conclusions?
3. How were data selected and arranged? What logic was used? Inductive? Deductive?
4. What name is given to this present state in light of the client-in-context story?

Framing

1. What theme emerged from the client's story? How?
2. What present state does the theme suggest?
3. Given the present state, what outcome is suggested?
4. How does concurrent consideration of outcome state, present state, and frame lead to specification of outcome criteria and test?
5. What outcome state is a logical consequence or contrast given the present-state information?
6. What is the client's keystone issue?

---

continued

Outcome State

    1. What influence does the frame have on the outcome state?

    2. What criteria indicate outcome achievement?

Present State

    1. What influence does the frame have on the present state?

    2. What test does the juxtaposition or contrast of outcome state with present state create?

Test

    1. What test conditions can be created?

    2. What is the test? What evidence is derived from the test conditions?

    3. How can test results be used to make clinical judgments?

Decision Making (Interventions)

    1. What nursing actions are necessary to achieve outcomes?

    2. How do nursing actions or clinical decisions promote achievement of the outcome state?

    3. How do interventions and decision making influence evidence derived from testing?

Judgment

    1. What do the test results mean?

    2. How does the judgment influence reflection?

    3. How does judgment influence decision making?

    4. How do judgment, reflection, and decision making influence reframing?

    5. How does this situation add to my clinical reasoning knowledge base?

By writing each element on the worksheet, it is easy to see how parts of the model relate to each other. As seen in Figure 5-1, on the far right-hand side, there is space to write the client's story. This space is called the client-in-context. It is a place for you to make notes and jot down relevant facts of the story. Moving to the left, there are places to write down inferences and conclusions that result from your logic and analysis of the facts. Remember, cue logic is the use of inductive and deductive thinking skills.

In the center and background of the worksheet are places for you to indicate the frame or theme that best represents the background issues regarding your thinking about the client story. The frame is the theme that often emerges after you have created a clinical reasoning web. The frame helps organize the present state, outcome state, and tests that you will structure. Decision making and reflection surround the framing. Remember, you think of many things simultaneously, and should use your reflective self to monitor your thinking and do reflection checks. At the center of the sheet are spaces for you to place the present state and outcome state side by side.

OPT Model Worksheet

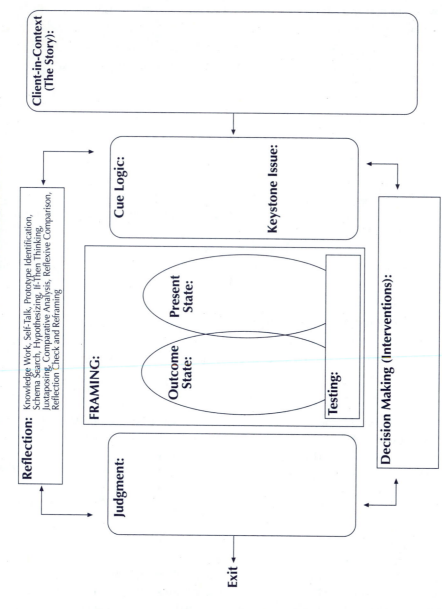

FIGURE 5-1 The OPT Model Worksheet

Putting the two states together in this way naturally shows where you are and where you want to be in terms of the client's care. The gap between where the client is and where you want the client to be is one way to create a test. Clinical decisions are choices you make about interventions. What decisions need to be made to help the client make the transition from her or his present state to a desired outcome state?

The reflection box is a reminder of the thinking strategies you can use to think about the client situation. These strategies also help make explicit many of the relationships among ideas and issues associated with the client's problems. Finally, the clinical judgment space on the far left-hand side of the paper is a place to write the results of the conclusions drawn from a test. Based on your comparison of where the client is and where you want the client to be, there is an evidence gap. Once you get evidence that fills that gap you need to make some sense of the evidence. What does it mean? Clinical judgments are all about the meaning you attribute to the evidence derived from the gap analysis of present to desired state.

Once you have experiences with clients, they become a part of your clinical reasoning learning history. Your experience adds to your schemas and informs your future thinking with clients who are similar to those with whom you have had experiences. Another action may be to reframe the situation and establish a new outcome state, present state, test, or set of intervention decisions. Follow along as we illustrate the use of the OPT Model Worksheet with an example.

The reasoning challenge begins with a description and understanding of the client's story. Consider these questions as a place to start: What is the story? How are cues related? What themes emerge? What is my outcome given the facts? What is the client's present state? What is the gap between the present state and desired outcome? What evidence will fill the gap? What kind of test can I create to obtain the evidence I need to make a clinical judgment? What clinical decisions will help me move the client from the present to the desired state? These questions help one become explicit about the thinking strategies embedded in the reasoning task. While the OPT Model Worksheet helps organize specific content and structure reasoning, another tool to facilitate the analysis and understanding of the multiple issues that are a part of the client's story is the Clinical Reasoning Web.

Clinical Reasoning Web

Client stories are complex. But with a little analysis, complex stories can be simplified into key issues. Spinning and weaving a web is the process of using thinking strategies to analyze and synthesize functional relationships among diagnostic hypotheses associated with a client's health status. A Clinical Reasoning Web is a useful tool in this simplification process. A Clinical Reasoning Web is a pictorial representation of the functional relationships among diagnostic hypotheses derived from the systems thinking that results in a convergence and identification of keystone issues that require nursing care. One way to begin reasoning is to spin and weave a web of relationships among identified nursing diagnoses associated with a medical condition.

Our experience is that many students begin care planning with the client's medical diagnosis in mind. Thus, it is a useful place to start. Once one considers the medical diagnosis, one can determine the nursing care consequences associated with the medical diagnosis. The steps to the creation of a Clinical Reasoning Web are described below.

To create a web, place the client's primary medical diagnosis in the middle of an 8-1/2 × 11 piece of paper. Second, generate possible nursing diagnoses that would be a consequence of the particular medical diagnosis for the client. Third, list the defining characteristics or cues displayed by the client for each nursing diagnosis you have identified. Fourth, reflect on the total picture on the paper and begin to draw lines of relationship, connection, or association among the nursing diagnoses. As you draw the lines, state to yourself your reasons for connecting these diagnoses. Fifth, determine which pattern has the highest priority for care and most efficiently and effectively represents the keystone nursing care needs of the client. Sixth, look once again at the sets of relationships and determine the theme that summarizes the client-in-context or the client's story.

Figure 5-2 is an example of a completed Clinical Reasoning Web for a person who had a medical diagnosis of chronic obstructive pulmonary disease (COPD).

Around the outer edges of the web are nursing diagnoses that were derived as consequences associated with the medical diagnosis. In this example, under each diagnosis are two to three cues or supporting evidence for the diagnosis. The bidirectional arrows that create the web effect are functional relationships between and among the nursing diagnosis possibilities. As one can see, there are many more arrows converging on the right-hand side of the diagram around the issues of ineffective breathing pattern, activity intolerance, fatigue, and self-care deficit. A keystone issue for this client is ineffective breathing. Keystone issues are one or more central supporting elements of the client's story that guide reasoning and care planning based on an analysis and synthesis of diagnostic possibilities as represented in a Clinical Reasoning Web.

The keystone issue contributes to the framing of the reasoning task. The frame serves as the backdrop for creating the present state, outcome state, and test conditions. Frame is to background as outcome, present state, and test are to foreground and figure in a Gestalt psychology perceptual illusion. For example, perhaps you have seen the Gestalt image of two faces staring at each other? The image can resemble two faces or a vase depending on your gaze. Another example would be the picture that appears as either an old hag or a young woman depending on your gaze. A Clinical Reasoning Web is a useful tool to help you in the reasoning process and is a way to represent some of the concurrent thinking in the OPT model.

To illustrate the way these tools and the OPT model work we now consider a case study. Before you begin the analysis of the case study, review the "big picture" relationships among critical thinking, reflective clinical reasoning and the thinking strategies listed in Table 5-1.

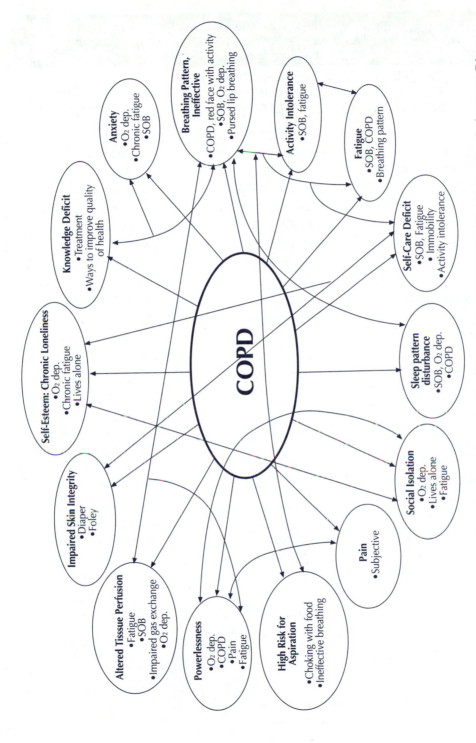

FIGURE 5-2 Completed Clinical Reasoning Web for a Client with (COPD) Chronic Obstructive Pulmonary Disease.

TABLE 5-1   The "Big Picture": Relationships among Critical Thinking, Reflective Clinical Reasoning, and Thinking Strategies

CRITICAL THINKING SKILLS	REFLECTIVE CLINICAL REASONING	THINKING STRATEGIES
Interpretation	Knowledge work	reading
categorize	Clinical vocabulary	memorizing
decode sentences	classification systems	drilling
clarify meaning	(e.g., NANDA, Gordon,	writing
	Omaha, *DSM-IV,* NIC,	reviewing research
	NOC)	practicing
Analysis	Cue logic	self-talk
examine ideas	cue connection	schema search
identify arguments	induction	prototype identification
analyze arguments	deduction	hypothesizing
	retroduction	
Inference	Framing	schema search
query evidence	cue connection	prototype identification
conjecture alternatives	scenario development	hypothesizing
draw conclusions	outcome specification	if–then thinking
	test creation	
Explanation	Decision making	schema search
state results	interventions	prototype identification
justify procedures	alternatives	comparative analysis
present arguments	consequences	if–then thinking
Evaluation	Testing	juxtaposition
assess claims	conduct test	comparative analysis
assess arguments	evaluate	revlexive comparison
Self-regulation	Judgment	reframing
self-examination	attribute meaning to	reflection check
self-correction	the test outcome	
(Facione & Facione,	frame new situation	
1996, p. 130)	create new test	

CASE STUDY: MR. RICHARD SMITH'S STORY

The combination of nursing classification systems, the OPT model, the Clinical Reasoning Web, and the OPT Model Worksheet are the essential ingredients for effective clinical reasoning. We illustrate this point below with a clinical case. From the initial story, we spin and weave a Clinical Reasoning Web and use the OPT Model Worksheet to organize our reasoning about the case study. Consider the story of Mr. Richard Smith.

Mr. Smith is a 56-year-old widower who was brought to the emergency room by EMS for what appears to be an acute case of dyspnea. He states that he awakened suddenly from sleep with severe shortness of breath (dyspnea). He tried to use his nebulizer treatment, but it did not help. In fact, his condition worsened. Mr. Smith said with a panicked, desperate expression, "It's so hard to breathe . . . can't catch my breath." He reports that he smoked one to two packs a day for 36 years but stopped smoking three months ago after a second sister died of lung cancer. His sisters were smokers for many years with a long history of acute bronchitis and emphysema. Currently, Mr. Smith has a medical diagnosis of emphysema and possible cor pulmonale. Examination and assessment revealed the following: nonproductive cough, decreased mental acuity; extreme shortness of breath with activity; fatigues easily; nonverbal expression of anxiety/fear, such as moderate sweating, trembling, irritability, and restlessness; extremities mildly cyanotic and cool to the touch; capillary refill sluggish ($\geq$ 4 seconds); greatly concerned that what happened to his two sisters might happen to him; worried about losing his job of 30 years due to too many sick days; children grown and live out of state; lives with teenage granddaughter who is 15 years old and 4 months pregnant. Vital signs: B/P 178/96, pulse 110, respirations 36/min (labored, irregular rhythm), and temperature 100.1. Blood gases: pH 7.36, O_2 sat 87%, $PaCO_2$ 48 mmHg, and HCO_3 24 mEq/L. He has limited health insurance/benefits.

Spinning and Weaving the Web

Mr. Smith presents in the ER with a history of emphysema and acute dyspnea. A review of the story allows us to use the cues to spin and weave the web. Putting emphysema with acute dyspnea in the center of the web allows one to generate multiple potential nursing diagnoses. Reflecting on the story suggests the following diagnostic hypotheses: ineffective breathing, impaired gas exchange, anxiety, fear, sleep pattern disturbance, activity intolerance, fatigue, altered health maintenance, at risk for infection, and noncompliance. Data about these hypotheses were derived from the story and are listed in Table 5-2.

Begin the development of a Clinical Reasoning Web for Mr. Smith with the medical condition in the center and the nursing diagnoses around the outer edges. (See Figure 5-3.)

The next step is to draw lines among nursing diagnoses that are related. For example, there is an obvious relationship between ineffective breathing pattern and anxiety. In

TABLE 5-2   Diagnostic Hypotheses and Client Cues from Mr. Richard Smith's Story

DIAGNOSTIC HYPOTHESES	CLIENT CUES
Ineffective breathing	Dyspnea, shortness of breath, respirations 36 per minute, irregular breathing rhythm, verbalization of "I can't breathe"
Impaired gas exchange	Dyspnea, confusion, ABG: pH 7.3 6, O_2 sat 87%, $PaCO_2$ 48 mmHg, HCO_3 24 mEq/L
Anxiety	Increased tension, apprehension, fearful, distressed, jittery, shakiness, fear of consequences, restlessness, trembling, sweating
Fear	Fear of dying like his sisters
Sleep pattern disturbance	Verbal complaints of waking up, restlessness
Activity intolerance	Verbal reports of fatigue and weakness, dyspnea, increased blood pressure
Fatigue	Verbal report of fatigue, inability to maintain normal routine, irritable, decreased performance
Altered health maintenance	History of lack of health-seeking behavior, expressed interest in improving health behaviors, reported lack of resources such as limited health insurance benefits
Ineffective management of therapeutic regimen	Condition worsened, verbalized difficulty with using nebulizer
At risk for infection	Decrease in ciliary action, stasis of body fluids, in nonproductive cough, chronic disease
Hyperthermia	Temperature of 100.1, increased respiratory rate (36), increased pulse rate (110)

addition, ineffective breathing suggests impaired gas exchange. In fact, impaired gas exchange may be the etiology of the anxiety. The reasoning behind this is the fact that if one cannot breathe then one becomes anxious. There may be a relationship between ineffective management of therapeutic regimen and fear, just as there is a relationship between ineffective management of therapeutic regimen and sleep pattern disturbance. If Mr. Smith cannot manage the emphysema then he is fearful and unable to sleep. There is also an obvious relationship between hyperthermia and high risk for infection. He has many cues for high risk for infection and the hyperthermia indicates that one sign of infection is present.

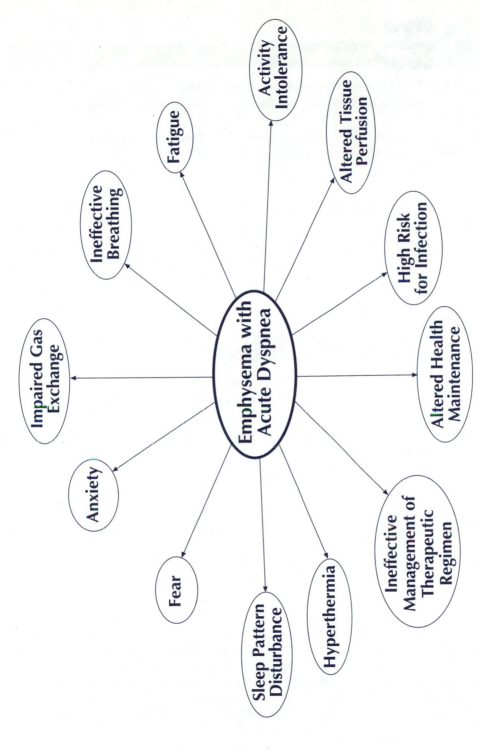

FIGURE 5-3 Beginning the Clinical Reasoning Web for Mr. Richard Smith

STOP AND THINK

1. **What do you think the relationships are among ineffective breathing pattern and altered tissue perfusion, impaired gas exchange, and fatigue?**
2. **What might be the relationship among altered tissue perfusion, high risk for infection, and hyperthermia?**

We know that if a person is not able to breathe properly, this leads to impaired gas exchange, which causes decrease in tissue perfusion, resulting in decreased oxygen consumption, which leads to increased fatigue and decreased activity tolerance. Looking at the functional relationships between and among these diagnoses, there are choices to be made. Look once again at the set of relationships that summarize the theme of the client-in-context story. (See Figure 5-4.)

STOP AND THINK

1. **What emerges as the focus of Mr. Smith's story?**
2. **What word or phrase would you use to describe this theme?**
3. **How does considering the total picture represented by the web help you think about the client from a multivariable or systems perspective?**

In this example, we have used the NANDA taxonomy to structure and give meaning to the cues. In the table specific cues are associated with each diagnosis and thus provide evidence for potential nursing diagnoses. Linking the diagnoses together in the web provides some direction for determining the present state for which nursing care will be developed. Data were selected both inductively and deductively based on the client's story and the knowledge of NANDA as the clinical vocabulary for clinical reasoning. In Figure 5-5 one can see the complexity of the reasoning involved.

Now that you have looked at the whole picture using the Clinical Reasoning Web, you are ready to use the OPT model and the OPT Model Worksheet to structure your thinking about the nursing care of Mr. Smith. As you think about Mr. Smith, you will concurrently consider the frame, outcome state, and present state. Each aspect of the OPT model contributes to the others. For example, based on Mr. Smith's story, one way to frame the situation is that he has fear and anxiety related to respiratory problems.

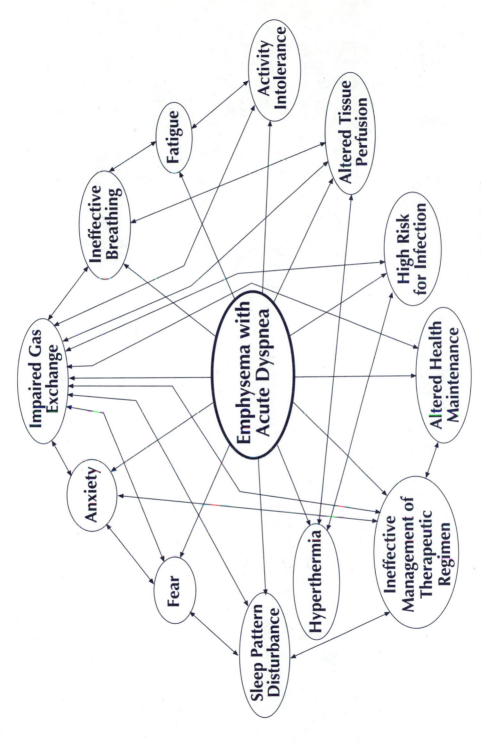

FIGURE 5-4 Developing Relationships in the Clinical Reasoning Web for Mr. Richard Smith

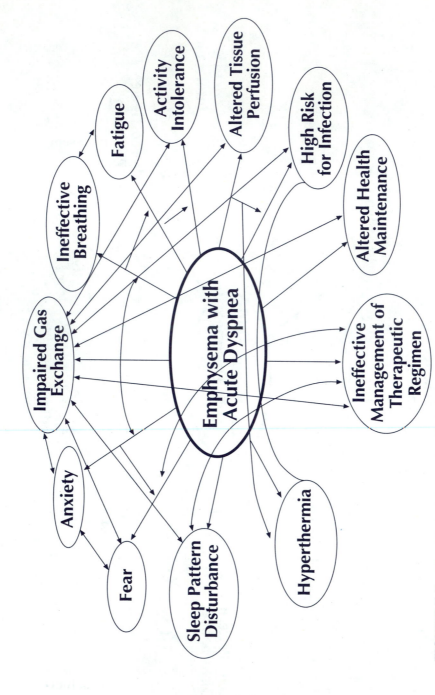

FIGURE 5-5 The Clinical Reasoning Web for Mr. Richard Smith

STOP AND THINK

1. **How did the theme emerge from the client's story?**
2. **What present state does the theme suggest?**
3. **Given the present state, what outcome is suggested?**
4. **How does concurrent consideration of outcome state, present state, and frame lead to specification of outcome criteria and test?**

Mr. Smith's respiratory problems become the focus for the juxtaposition and contrast of his present state with a desired outcome state. Based on an analysis of the relationships one way to name the present state is impaired gas exchange as evidenced by O_2 sat of 87 with cyanosis of extremities. As a result of identifying the present state as impaired gas exchange, a logical consequence and juxtaposition for a well-formed outcome is an O_2 sat of 92 with no cyanosis.

STOP AND THINK

1. **What influence does the frame have on the outcome state?**
2. **What criteria indicate outcome achievement?**
3. **What test does the juxtaposition of outcome state and present state create?**

Given the frame of fear and anxiety related to respiratory problems and the present state of impaired gas exchange as evidenced by O_2 sat of 87 and a desired outcome state of 92%, we have the basic elements of the test. The test is the comparison of blood gas values, signs, and symptoms at a predetermined time following nursing interventions.

STOP AND THINK

1. **What nursing actions are necessary for outcome achievement?**
2. **How do nursing actions or clinical decisions promote achievement of outcome state?**

Several nursing actions or decisions are possible to achieve the desired outcome. These include oxygen therapy, education about pursed-lip breathing, bronchodilator therapy, positioning, and monitoring vital signs. All of these interventions will have a direct effect on impaired gas exchange and will assist the client in making the transition from the initial present state to desired outcome state. Mr. Smith's present state also includes fear and anxiety about his inability to breath as well as fear and anxiety about his ability to continue to function in all his roles. The interventions listed above will have a direct effect on the acute fear and anxiety. The interventions will not influence the continuing fear and anxiety associated with the consequences of his chronic medical condition. An additional intervention to treat the fear and anxiety is therapeutic communication.

STOP AND THINK

1. **What test conditions can be created?**
2. **What is done to conduct the test?**
3. **How can test results be used to make clinical judgments?**

When you conduct a test by juxtaposing the present state and outcome state, there are three possible consequences. First, Mr. Smith could achieve and match the desired outcome state of 92% without cyanosis and accompanying signs and symptoms. Second, Mr. Smith's condition could deteriorate while under your nursing care. This situation would change the story and activate the cue logic and result in reframing of the situation and lead to a different present state, outcome state, and test. Third, Mr. Smith could improve but not achieve or meet the desired outcome. You will need to reflect on this situation and determine why it has occurred and institute new decisions or interventions to promote the transition to the outcome state. The consequences of these tests are the data one uses to make clinical judgments. Clinical judgments are the meanings that are attributed to test results. The concurrent consideration of test results, judgment, reflection, and decision making determine if continued clinical reasoning is required or if the nurse can move on to another task.

STOP AND THINK

1. **What do the test results mean?**
2. **How does the judgment influence reflection?**
3. **How does judgment influence decision making?**
4. **How do judgment, reflection, and decision making influence reframing?**

The results of the test were that Mr. Smith had O_2 sat of 92 or greater without cyanosis, unlabored respirations of 18, and a verbal report of decreased dyspnea. Therefore, outcome was achieved. What these results mean in terms of clinical judgment suggest that the decisions and nursing actions that were initiated were effective in transitioning Mr. Smith from the present state to the outcome state. If the test had revealed an O_2 sat of 87, the judgment would be very different. The nurse would need to institute more aggressive interventions or reframe the situation to reflect the new condition relying on the addition of new cues.

THINKING STRATEGIES THAT SUPPORT REFLECTIVE CLINICAL REASONING

One of the essential parts of the OPT model is reflection. Some of the components of reflection are self-monitoring, self-evaluation, and self-correction. Thinking about your thinking helps you evaluate, discover flaws in your thinking, and correct your clinical reasoning skills. Thinking strategies are specific reflection techniques that nurses use when engaged in reflective clinical reasoning. Becoming aware of the specific thinking strategies you use to support reflective clinical reasoning and the use of the OPT model will help you develop critical thinking or, as Facione and Facione (1996) define it, "purposeful self-regulatory judgment which results in interpretation, analysis, evaluation, and inference as well as the explanation of the evidential, conceptual, methodological, criteriological or contextual considerations upon which that judgment was based" (p. 36).

Knowledge Work

Clinical reasoning presupposes that you have done the knowledge work of reading, memorizing, drilling, writing, reviewing of research, and practicing. This knowledge work is necessary to gain the clinical vocabulary of the classification system in order to interpret data about the client-in-context. It would have been very difficult to generate diagnostic hypotheses for Mr. Smith if one did not know the definitions and classifications of impaired gas exchange, impaired breathing pattern, and so on. Other fundamental knowledge needed to plan care for Mr. Smith includes information about physiological, psychological, and sociological functioning. Fundamental knowledge in these areas are such things as normal and abnormal blood gas values, vital signs, and the psychodynamics of anxiety and fear. Fundamental knowledge in these areas helped one interpret, analyze, explain, and infer what was going on with Mr. Smith. Several other thinking strategies supported clinical reasoning. The thinking strategies of self-talk, schema search, prototype identification, hypothesizing, if–then thinking, comparative analysis, juxtaposing, and decision making (reflexive comparison, reframing, and reflection check) are defined and described below.

Self-Talk

Self-talk is the process of expressing one's thoughts to one's self. Self-talk answers the question, "What are the nursing diagnostic possibilities associated with the medical condition of emphysema?" The answer to this question results in the identification of the diagnostic hypotheses relevant to the case. For example, the human responses to emphysema include such things as ineffective breathing pattern, impaired gas exchange, fatigue, anxiety, and fear. Self-talk also is useful when spinning and weaving the Clinical Reasoning Web. One has to think out loud and reason about the possible relationships and connections among diagnostic hypotheses. For example, self-talk stimulates questions about relationships among nursing diagnoses. We asked the question, "What are the relationships among ineffective breathing pattern, impaired gas exchange, fatigue, and anxiety?"

Prototype Identification

Prototype identification is using a model case as a reference point for comparative analysis. Mr. Smith represents one instance of a client with emphysema. Knowing what the prototypical client with emphysema in an acute crisis is likely to exhibit serves as a standard. With prototype identification, you use the textbook case of emphysema in acute distress as the standard and reference point for comparative analysis.

Schema Search

Schema search is the process of accessing general and/or specific patterns of past experiences that might apply to the current situation. The reason that students like a lot of clinical experiences is because these experiences help them build schema. Past clinical experiences are helpful in reasoning about a specific case. One way to develop expertise is to use self-talk as you build schema. Each experience you have with a client creates a web in your mind. The more experiences you have, the more complex the web and the easier it is to access. Novices are in the process of spinning and weaving memory webs with each clinical experience. Experts have multiple webs superimposed on one another. That is why they can reason about situations so effectively and quickly. Consider the web and the associations you made with Mr. Smith in the case study. You now have a schema for a client experiencing respiratory distress. The schema includes what this client exhibited, what interventions were done, and what the outcomes were. These memories become the foundation for clinical reasoning expertise.

Hypothesizing

Hypothesizing is determining an explanation that accounts for a set of facts that can be tested by further investigation. Hypothesizing presupposes use and understanding of clinical vocabulary. Given Mr. Smith's story, we tried to explain the set of facts he shared in the context of his emergency room visit. These explanations were called diagnostic hypotheses. They are guesses about what might explain his situation, such as high risk for infection, hyperthermia, and ineffective management of therapeutic regime. We also hypothesized that self-care deficit and altered health care maintenance might be issues to be considered. However, when we tested self-care deficit as a hypothesis, it was not supported by the data.

The diagnostic hypotheses become the origins and insertion points for making associations when one develops a Clinical Reasoning Web. Hypothesizing includes if–then thinking; however, it is a more formal statement or declaration about how specifically sets of facts are related. Hypothesis testing requires gathering of evidence under controlled conditions to affirm or negate the proposed relationship. As we begin spinning and weaving the web, we generated a number of diagnostic hypotheses. Once nursing diagnoses were identified, it was easier to see how these diagnoses might be related through hypothesizing.

If–Then Thinking

If–then thinking involves linking ideas and consequences together in a logical sequence. In Mr. Smith's case, ineffective breathing pattern was linked to an increase in anxiety. Doesn't it make sense that if he had difficulty breathing then he would become anxious? Another example of if–then thinking links impaired gas exchange with fatigue. If Mr. Smith was not adequately oxygenated, then he would not have adequate tissue perfusion. If Mr. Smith's tissues were not perfused, then he would not have the energy necessary for activities. Thus, his lack of energy is made evident by symptoms of fatigue that are a consequence of impaired gas exchange. Much of clinical reasoning involves linking ideas and consequences together in a logical sequence.

Comparative Analysis

Comparative analysis is a thinking strategy that involves considering the strengths and weaknesses of competing alternatives. Once diagnostic hypotheses and their relationships are made explicit using the web, comparative analysis is used to determine which of these relationships is the keystone or the central supporting issues of Mr. Smith's situation. Identifying the keystone issues enables the nurse to focus care. Once a keystone issue is identified, it has a domino effect. Once we take care of Mr. Smith's impaired gas exchange, we influence his tissue perfusion, breathing pattern, activity intolerance, fatigue, anxiety, and fear.

Juxtaposing

Juxtaposing is another essential thinking skill. Juxtaposing involves putting the present state condition next to the outcome state. The side-by-side contrast of one state with the other illustrates the differences between the two states. The differences or gaps evident from the present to desired state help establish the conditions for the creation of a test in the OPT model. Given Mr. Smith's initial blood gas of 87% and the desired blood gas of 92% a contrast or side-by-side comparison of these two values, 92% and 87%, creates a test. There is a gap that must be bridged from one state to the other. In order to meet or match the desired outcome criteria of O_2 sat. of 92%, Mr. Smith needs to increase his blood gas oxygen saturation value at least 5 percentage points. Juxtaposing enables one to set up essential elements between two states. Decisions one makes and interventions one initiates help bridge the gap between juxtaposed conditions.

Using NIC, the knowledge contained in the intervention categories assists in decision making about interventions needed to transition Mr. Smith to his desired state. NIC is a knowledge classification system that provides guidance concerning activities and interventions nurses use to help clients make the transition from identified present states to specified outcomes states. The nurse must decide among an array of possible interventions. Part IV of NIC (McCloskey & Bulechek, 1996) provides a resource that links NIC interventions to NANDA diagnoses. Given the present state of impaired gas exchange, nursing interventions that will help transition Mr. Smith to his desired outcome state include respiratory monitoring (which includes such activities as monitoring for changes in ABG values as appropriate), respiratory treatments, anxiety reduction, calming techniques, emotional support, and energy management. These nursing interventions are among the many choices or clinical decisions that the nurse makes to transition Mr. Smith from his present state to the desired outcome state.

Decision Making (Interventions)

Decision making is the process of making choices about nursing actions. Decision making is based on the compilation of nursing interventions as categorized in the knowledge classification system as set forth by NIC.

The nurse applies reflection and reasoning to decide that the intervention will be the most effective in bringing about the desired outcome. The thinking strategies of reflexive comparison, reframing, and reflection check will help guide the reasoning process.

Reflexive Comparison

Reflexive comparison is a thinking strategy that involves constant comparison of the client's state from time of observation to time of observation. For example, each time blood gas values on Mr. Smith are reviewed, the nurse will compare Mr. Smith's progress from one observation to the next. In this way the nurse is using Mr. Smith as his own standard in terms of making progress toward the desired outcome state and target blood gas level. Review Figure 5-6, a completed OPT Model Worksheet for Mr. Smith. Consider how all the parts of the model fit together before you go on to the next section about reframing.

Reframing

Reframing is the thinking strategy of attributing a different meaning to the content or context of a situation given a set of cues, tests, decisions, and judgments. Once Mr. Smith reaches his desired level of blood gas values and impaired gas exchange is resolved, it may become evident that his anxiety and fear are not resolved. Remember, clinical reasoning is reflective, concurrent, creative, and critical thinking embedded in nursing practice that nurses use to frame, juxtapose, and test the match between a client's present state and desired outcome state. It may be that one needs to reframe Mr. Smith's keystone issue. The challenge now becomes helping Mr. Smith transition from his states of anxiety and fear to calm and confidence. Another way to

OPT Model Worksheet

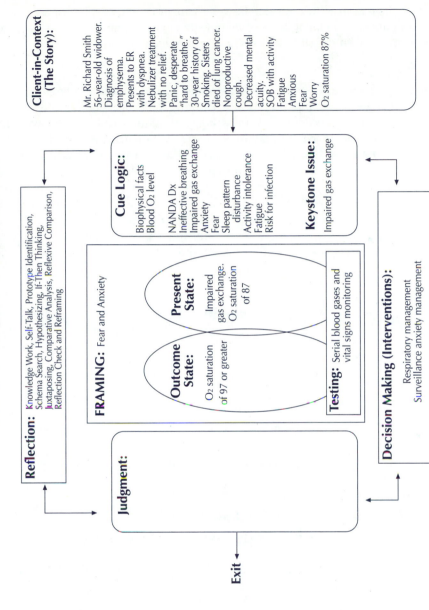

Client-in-Context (The Story):

Mr. Richard Smith 56-year-old widower. Diagnosis of emphysema. Presents to ER with dyspnea. Nebulizer treatment with no relief. Panic, desperate "hard to breathe." 30-year history of Smoking. Sisters died of lung cancer. Nonproductive cough. Decreased mental acuity. SOB with activity Fatigue Anxious Fear Worry O₂ saturation 87%

Reflection: Knowledge Work, Self-Talk, Prototype Identification, Schema Search, Hypothesizing, If-Then Thinking, Juxtaposing, Comparative Analysis, Reflexive Comparison, Reflection Check and Reframing

Cue Logic:

Biophysical facts
Blood O₂ level

NANDA Dx
Ineffective breathing
Impaired gas exchange
Anxiety
Fear
Sleep pattern disturbance
Activity intolerance
Fatigue
Risk for infection

Keystone Issue:

Impaired gas exchange

FRAMING: Fear and Anxiety

Outcome State:
O₂ saturation of 97 or greater

Present State:
Impaired gas exchange. O₂ saturation of 87

Testing: Serial blood gases and vital signs monitoring

Decision Making (Interventions):
Respiratory management
Surveillance anxiety management

Judgment:

Exit

FIGURE 5-6 Completed OPT Model Worksheet for Mr. Richard Smith

reframe the situation is to consider how he can more effectively manage his own therapeutic regime. Reframing is the thinking strategy that enables one to attribute different meaning given the story and context and reflection on the situation.

Reflection Check

A reflection check involves reflecting and analyzing the critical and creative thinking skills and strategies that support clinical reasoning. Reflection check is the process of self-monitoring, self-correcting, self-reinforcing, and self-evaluating one's own thinking about a specific task or situation (Herman, Pesut, & Conard, 1994; Pesut & Herman, 1992; Worrell, 1990). A reflection check pinpoints all that you have done correctly, it also identifies errors and provides an opportunity to understand how to fix them. A reflection check involves understanding how the critical thinking skills identified by Facione and Facione (1996) support reflective clinical reasoning through the use of specific thinking strategies. Return to Table 5-1 The "Big Picture": Relationships among Critical Thinking, Reflective Clinical Reasoning, and Thinking Strategies, and consider Mr. Smith as you review the critical thinking and reasoning you used in Mr. Smith's case.

STOP AND THINK

1. **Have I interpreted Mr. Smith's case correctly?**
2. **Am I satisfied with my analysis of ideas and arguments?**
3. **Have I made appropriate inferences, conjectures, and conclusions based on the evidence available?**
4. **Are my explanations sound in terms of result, procedures, and arguments?**
5. **Are the claims and arguments for conducting and evaluating the test sound?**
6. **How would an expert nurse perceive this situation?**
7. **What corrective measures do I need to take?**
8. **Explain how past clinical experiences influenced your reasoning about this case.**
9. **How will experience with this case influence future clinical reasoning given clients with a similar story?**

Thinking Strategies Worksheet

We have provided the Thinking Strategies Worksheet to help you master the thinking skills that support reflective clinical reasoning. Apply your study skills and identify instances of each of the thinking strategies based on the analysis presented about Mr. Smith's case. Complete the Thinking Strategies worksheet in Table 5-3.

TABLE 5-3   Thinking Strategies Worksheet

THINKING STRATEGY	DEFINITION OF THE STRATEGY	EXAMPLE FROM MR. SMITH'S CASE
Knowledge Work	Active use of reading, memorizing, drilling, writing, reviewing research, and practicing to learn clinical vocabulary	
Self-Talk	Expressing one's thoughts to one's self	
Schema Search	Accessing general and/or specific patterns of past experiences that might apply to the current situation	
Prototype Identification	Using a model case as a reference point for comparative analysis	
Hypothesizing	Determining an explanation that accounts for a set of facts that can be tested by further investigation	
If–Then Thinking	Linking ideas and consequences together in a logical sequence	
Comparative Analysis	Considering the strengths and weaknesses of competing alternatives	
Juxtaposing	Putting the present state condition next to the outcome state in a side-by-side contrast	
Reflexive Comparison	Constantly comparing the client's state from time of observation to time of observation	
Reframing	Attributing a different meaning to the content or context of a situation based on tests, decisions, or judgments	
Reflection Check	Self-examination and self-correction of critical thinking skills and thinking strategies that support clinical reasoning	

SUMMARY

Knowledge work requires both content and structure. Knowledge is contained in the classification systems and is continuing to be developed through practice experiences and research. The OPT model provides the structure for clinical reasoning. We introduced three tools to assist you in putting the OPT model to use: the OPT Model Worksheet, Clinical Reasoning Web, and Thinking Strategies Worksheet. We illustrated how these tools were used with an example of a man in the emergency room. Thinking strategies that supported reflective clinical reasoning were defined and described with examples from the case study. We discussed the reflection check as a thinking strategy to help you self-monitor, self-evaluate, and self-correct thinking. The reflection check enables one to understand how critical and creative thinking skills and strategies are supportive of reflective clinical reasoning. We concluded the chapter with a challenge exercise related to mastering the thinking strategies and their definitions by associating them with examples from the case study. The learning tools introduced in this chapter serve as the foundation for reasoning about client cases across various contexts. The next chapters of the book will introduce client cases in the contexts of primary care, acute care, community health care, community mental health care, and long-term care.

KEY CONCEPTS

1. Knowledge work requires content, structure, and reasoning skills.
2. Nursing knowledge classification systems provide the content for clinical reasoning.
3. The OPT model provides the structure for clinical reasoning.
4. The OPT Model Worksheet provides a graphic representation of the structure of the OPT model and is a guide to the thinking that occurs when using the OPT model.
5. Structured questions for the OPT Model Worksheet serve as a guide for clinical reasoning.
6. The Clinical Reasoning Web is both a strategy and learning tool that facilitates reasoning about functional relationships between and among nursing diagnoses.
7. Novices spin and weave memory webs with each clinical experience, which helps them with future care of clients with similar stories.
8. The study skills of reading, memorizing, drilling, writing, reviewing, and practicing support the acquisition of clinical vocabulary.
9. The thinking strategies of self-talk, schema search, prototype identification, hypothesizing, if–then thinking, comparative analysis, juxtaposing, and decision making, reflexive comparison, reframing, and reflection check foster development of critical thinking and reflective clinical reasoning.

10. Using nursing knowledge classification systems, the OPT Model Worksheet, the Clinical Reasoning Web, and the Thinking Strategies Worksheet enables one to reason more effectively.

STUDY QUESTIONS AND ACTIVITIES

1. Brainstorm with classmates on how you can learn the clinical vocabulary associated with several of the nursing knowledge classification systems.

2. Once you have received your next clinical assignment, use a Clinical Reasoning Web to map out relationships and issues after you talk with your client and listen to his or her story. Use the OPT Model Worksheet to organize the results of your web.

3. Compare and contrast reasoning using the OPT model and the traditional nursing process.

List any questions you had as you were using the OPT model. Talk with your instructor or another classmate about your questions. Together can you find the answers?

REFERENCES

Facione, N. C., & Facione, P. A., (1996). Externalizing the critical thinking in knowledge development and clinical judgment. *Nursing Outlook, 44*(3), 129–136.

Herman, J. A., Pesut, D. J., & Conard, L. (1994). Using metacognitive skills: The quality audit. *Nursing Diagnosis, 5*(2), 55–64.

McCloskey, J. C., & Bulechek, G. (1996). *Nursing intervention classification* (2nd ed.). St. Louis, MO: Mosby.

North American Nursing Diagnosis Association. (1996). *Nursing diagnoses: Definitions and classifications 1997–1998*. Philadelphia, PA: North American Nursing Diagnosis Association.

Pesut, D. J., & Herman, J. A. (1992). Metacognitive skills in diagnostic reasoning. *Nursing Diagnosis, 3*(4), 148–154.

Pesut, D. J., Herman, J. A., & Fowler, L. P. (1997). Toward a revolution in thinking: The OPT model of clinical reasoning. In J. McCloskey & H. Grace (Eds.), *Current issues in nursing* (5th ed., pp. 88–92). St. Louis, MO: Mosby.

Worrell, P. (1990). Metacognition: Implications for instruction in nursing education. *Journal of Nursing Education, 29*, 170–175.

CHAPTER 6

Clinical Reasoning with a Wellness Focus: Primary Care and Marjory Gordon's Functional Health Patterns

COMPETENCIES

After completing this chapter, the reader should be able to:

1. Discuss the importance of primary health care for health promotion and disease prevention.

2. Identify 21 priority health care needs for the nation.

3. Apply the OPT model to a primary care client case study.

4. Spin and weave a Clinical Reasoning Web based on a primary care case study.

5. Develop an OPT Model Worksheet for a primary care client.

6. Use the Thinking Strategies Worksheet to identify strategies for cue logic, framing, testing, reflection, clinical decision making, and clinical judgment in the case study scenario.

7. Explain the reflection checks that support clinical reasoning in this case.

8. Explain how reasoning about the clinical case study influences future reasoning about clients in a primary care context.

INTRODUCTION

The purpose of this chapter and several that follow is to explore selected health care issues and needs of clients in specific health care contexts. Contexts vary, but clinical reasoning across contexts is similar. The OPT model provides structure for reasoning in any context given the facts and stories of individual client cases. In this chapter, we focus on wellness. Maintaining and enhancing health is what primary care is all about. We highlight some of the issues regarding priority areas for the nation's health status. We identify 21 priority areas for health promotion, and disease prevention. Registered professional nurses are the health coaches of the future. A nurse's knowledge base supports wellness, health promotion, and disease prevention. Given the nation's emphasis on primary care, nurses who advocate health behavior and take their roles as health educators seriously are likely to be in great demand.

The OPT model can be used to structure reasoning about wellness objectives. In this chapter we introduce a case that is wellness-related. We demonstrate use of the Clinical Reasoning Web, OPT Model Worksheet, and Thinking Strategies Worksheet. Toward the end of the chapter we challenge you to review the case and to complete an OPT Model Worksheet and Thinking Strategies Worksheet so that you can exercise and evaluate your thinking and reasoning skills.

HEALTH CARE ISSUES AND NEEDS IN PRIMARY CARE

The concept of primary care is a logical foundation for an effective health care system. The goals of primary care are to keep people healthy. Keeping people healthy has ethical, economic, and health care consequences for society. Primary care is the foundation of an integrated health care system and is one strategy to achieve desired health outcomes (Donaldson, Yordy, Lohr, & Vanselow, 1996).

The United States Public Health Service developed a health agenda for the nation, Healthy People 2000. This document identifies health status objectives around 21 priority areas. The areas are clustered under the major headings of health promotion, health protection, preventive services, and surveillance.

The central purpose of Healthy People 2000 is to commit the nation to achieving three health related goals: an increased span of healthy life; reduced differences in health status among individuals and groups; and improved access to health care for all Americans. Health promotion strategies are those related to the personal lifestyle choices that people make regarding their health and health behaviors. People are capable of making healthy choices around the areas of physical activity, nutrition, smoking, alcohol, family planning, violence and/or abusive behavior. Encouraging people to develop good health habits is critical to meeting the health promotion objectives of the Healthy People initiative.

BOX 6-1   Healthy People 2000 Priority Areas

Health Promotion
1. Physical Activity and Fitness
2. Nutrition
3. Tobacco
4. Alcohol and Other Drugs
5. Family Planning
6. Mental Health and Mental Disorders
7. Violent and Abusive Behavior
8. Educational and Community-Based Programs

Health Protection
9. Unintentional Injuries
10. Occupational Safety and Health
11. Environmental Health
12. Food and Drug Safety
13. Oral Health

Preventive Services
14. Maternal and Infant Health
15. Heart Disease and Stroke
16. Cancer
17. Diabetes and Chronic Disabling Conditions
18. HIV Infection
19. Sexually Transmitted Diseases
20. Immunization and Infectious Diseases
21. Clinical Preventive Services

Surveillance and Data Systems
22. Surveillance and Data Systems

Another category of objectives is health protection. Health protection strategies are those related to environmental or regulatory measures that confer protection on large populations or groups. Interventions in this area are protective and health promotion-related. Often a community rather than an individual is the focus. Issues such as injuries, occupational safety and health, environmental health, oral health, and food and drug safety are the focus of concern. In addition, preventive services include counseling, screening, immunization, and drug intervention programs. Emphasis areas for preventive services include maternal/infant health as well as decreasing heart disease, stroke, cancer, diabetes, chronic disabling disease, HIV, and infectious diseases. Each of these health conditions is influenced through health promotion, protection, and preventive services. Surveillance and data systems to ensure a way to monitor progress in achievement of objectives is one of the last categories of objectives.

The goals and objectives are consistent with nursing approaches to wellness (Pender, 1996).Wellness involves attention to exercise, nutrition, and personal responsibility. While the goals and objectives of Healthy People 2000 are targets for the nation, each individual contributes to his or her personal health management plan. Personal health involves decisions about physical activity and fitness, nutrition management, abstinence from use of tobacco products and drugs, moderate use of alcohol, and risk reduction. Changing the health behavior of individuals, groups, and communities is no easy task (Pender, 1996). Futurists predict that health and wellness will be a major trend for the next decade. Lifestyle design, counseling, and coaching for health and wellness are projected to be big business and a large industry (Bezold & Mayer, 1996).

NURSING KNOWLEDGE IN PRIMARY CARE: GORDON'S FUNCTIONAL HEALTH PATTERNS

The OPT model provides the structure for clinical reasoning about health and wellness. Marjory Gordon's functional health pattern classification system enables nurses to quickly pinpoint health concerns in 11 functional areas. Gordon's functional health patterns provide a clinical vocabulary and content for clinical reasoning in primary care. According to Gordon, using the functional health patterns as an assessment guide enables one to quickly determine areas of strength and deviations from norms. Once a deviation is identified, one can zero in on the area and reason about the area's influence on health promotion and health maintenance efforts. Follow along as we use Gordon's functional health patterns as a way to assess and analyze the health care needs of a predominately well individual, Ms. Beth White.

CASE STUDY: MS. BETH WHITE'S STORY

Remember, reasoning challenges begin with the story about the client-in-context. Ms. Beth White is a 46-year-old engineer. She is married and has two children. She is very successful and works long hours (12 to 14 hours a day). She understands that she has personal responsibility for her own health. Recently she finds it difficult to do all she wants to do in regard to health maintenance and health-enhancing activities. She has a hectic schedule. There is a history of breast cancer in her family. Her father was recently diagnosed with dementia.

Ms. White is dedicated to her family. She enjoys being a mother and participating in activities with her family, which include concerts, ballet performances, and soccer games. She occasionally walks around her neighborhood, swims, and bikes with her children and husband.

Ms. White loves to cook, although she does not have the time or energy to plan and prepare meals as she would like. She is conscientious about preparing low-fat meals. She does not smoke and drinks moderately. She weighs 125 pounds and is 65 inches tall. She currently takes a multiple vitamin, a calcium supplement, and estrogen replacement therapy. She reports no problems with her bowel or bladder functions.

Ms. White is beginning to experience some of the signs of aging, including less flexibility, decreased visual acuity, decreased energy, and more difficulty controlling her weight. She has times when she is depressed and overwhelmed about her work situation. Recently, she has had trouble sleeping because she is worried about getting her work done. She gets up every day at 4:00 A.M. to catch up on office work. By 6:00 A.M. she is packing the children's lunches and getting everyone up for the day.

Over the past three months Ms. White has experienced increased stress at work, resulting in mood swings. She is struggling with conflicts related to her professional aspirations and her personal life as a wife and mother. In terms of her sexual and reproductive health status, she identifies limited opportunities for intimacy with her husband because of the ever vigilant presence of her children. She believes if you work hard, success will come your way. She feels she has to work harder than others because she is a woman in a predominately male profession.

Ms. White realizes the importance of maintaining her health and regular periodic health exams. Her office has a contract with a local HMO that provides annual health screening, which includes a physical exam, blood work, and health lifestyle appraisals. Her latest physical was within normal limits. Her lifestyle screening indicated she needed to learn more about stress management, exercise, and increasing her physical activity. Based on the results of her health appraisal, Ms. White makes an appointment with a nurse who is a health coach.

STOP AND THINK

1. **If you were Ms. White's health coach, how would you reason about her needs and care?**
2. **How might the OPT model assist you in structuring and reasoning about outcomes important in this case?**
3. **What cues are associated with her story?**
4. **Given the fact that Ms. White is fairly healthy, what can you build on to maximize wellness?**

SPINNING AND WEAVING THE CLINICAL REASONING WEB

As the nurse coach listens to Ms. White's story, the coach reviews data from her lifestyle assessment questionnaire, blood work, and physical exam. The nurse uses Gordon's functional health patterns as the taxonomy to structure and give meaning to the cues, as she connects ideas and issues in order to spin and weave a Clinical Reasoning Web.

STOP AND THINK

1. **How would you develop the cue logic associated with this story?**
2. **Which specific cues lead to present-state inferences or conclusions?**
3. **How are data selected and arranged?**
4. **What do you think the keystone issue is in this case?**
5. **What outcome is suggested by a review of the story?**

Listed in Table 6-1 are the functional health patterns, data from Ms. White's story, and diagnostic hypotheses that might be derived from the story and data.

Based on Ms. White's story, cue logic, and results from the health assessment questionnaire the nurse determines that activity and exercise is the keystone issue. As a consequence of inactivity, Ms. White's experiences fatigue, sleep pattern disturbance, depression, alteration in mood, ineffective coping, decreased intimacy, and altered nutrition. The frame is health-seeking behavior. How did the nurse arrive at these conclusions?

Both the frame and the keystone issue came from the process of developing the Clinical Reasoning Web. Remember how the web in the previous chapter was developed? The first step was to write the medical diagnosis in the middle of a piece of paper. Ms. White does not have a medical diagnosis. She is a healthy woman who wants to change her lifestyle so she can gain a higher level of wellness. It follows that the web begins with health maintenance as shown in Figure 6-1.

THINKING STRATEGIES THAT SUPPORT REFLECTIVE CLINICAL REASONING

Recall that clinical reasoning presupposes that you have done the reading, memorizing, drilling, writing, and practicing necessary to use the clinical vocabulary of the classification system of choice. For example, if one did not know the definitions,

TABLE 6-1 Health Patterns and Data from Ms. Beth White's Story

PATTERN	DATA	DIAGNOSTIC HYPOTHESES
Health perception/health management pattern—client's perceived pattern of health and well-being and how health is managed	Accepts personal responsibility for health, values periodic health screening and exams, uses health resources available to her	Health-seeking behaviors related to exercise, nutrition, and stress management
Nutritional/metabolic pattern—pattern of food and fluid consumption relative to metabolic need and pattern indicators of local nutrient supply	Prepares low-fat meals, enjoys cooking, takes vitamins and calcium supplements, more difficulty controlling weight	Altered nutrition—at risk for more than body requirements
Elimination pattern—patterns of excretory function (bowel, bladder, and skin)	No bowel or bladder problems	Functioning well
Activity/exercise pattern—pattern of exercise, activity, leisure, and recreation	Fatigue, less flexibility, decreased energy, walks, swims, bikes with children, values vigorous physical activity but limited by time and hectic schedule	Fatigue, alterations in physical activity and exercise
Sleep/rest pattern—patterns of sleep, rest, and relaxation	Wakes early, trouble sleeping	Sleep pattern disturbance
Cognitive/perceptual pattern—sensory-perceptual and cognitive pattern	Decreased visual acuity alterations	Sensory-perceptual
Self-perception/self-concept pattern—self-concept pattern and perceptions of self (e.g., body comfort, body image, feeling state)	Perceives self as successful, hardworking, competent, driven to work harder because she is in an all-male profession, sometimes gets depressed and overwhelmed	At risk for situational depression, alteration in moods

continued

TABLE 6-1 *(continued)*

PATTERN	DATA	DIAGNOSTIC HYPOTHESES
Role/relationship pattern—pattern of role-engagements and relationships	Conflicts related to professional aspirations and personal life	Role strain, alterations in family process
Sexuality/reproductive pattern—client's patterns of satisfaction and dissatisfaction with sexuality pattern; describes reproductive patterns	Intimacy with husband complicated by presence of children	Alterations in sexual activity
Coping/stress tolerance pattern—general coping pattern and effectiveness of the pattern in terms of stress tolerance	Feeling depressed and overwhelmed about her job situation, limited diversional activities	Potential ineffective coping related to stress
Value/belief pattern—pattern of values, beliefs (including spirtual), or goals that guide choices or decisions	Believes that if you work hard, success will come your way Committed to health enhancement	Health seeking behavior

classifications, and categories of diagnoses associated with Gordon's functional health patterns it would be difficult to pinpoint issues and deviations that benefit from intervention.

Other fundamental knowledge needed to plan care for Ms. White includes knowledge about physiological, psychological, and sociological functioning. Especially important knowledge is an understanding of the health outcomes of regular exercise. Knowledge in the areas of stress and coping is also important. Knowledge in these areas helps one to interpret, analyze, explain, and infer what is going on with Ms. White. The thinking strategies of self-talk, schema search, prototype identification, hypothesizing, and if–then thinking support reasoning as the Clinical Reasoning Web is developed. Let us examine and discuss each of these thinking strategies.

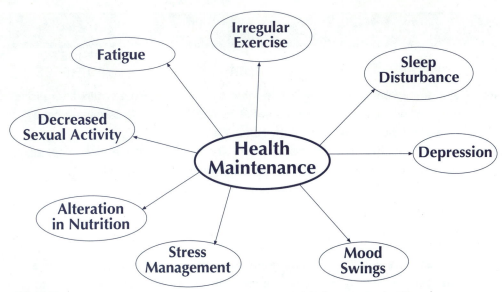

FIGURE 6-1   Beginning the Clinical Reasoning Web for Ms. Beth White

Self-Talk

Self-talk is the process of expressing one's thoughts to one's self. Self-talk answers the question, "What are the nursing diagnostic possibilities associated with Ms. White's story? The answer to this question results in the identification of relevant diagnostic hypotheses. For example, data from Ms. White's story indicate the following: fatigue, sleep pattern disturbance, depression, alteration in activity and exercise, alteration in nutrition, mood swings, decreased sexual activity, and stress management problems. Now add these hypotheses to the web by placing them around health maintenance. Figure 6-1 shows the web at this stage of development.

Continue to use if–then thinking to identify functional relationships among the possible diagnostic hypotheses for Ms. White. Stress management can be related to mood swings, depression, decreased sexual activity, and alteration in nutrition. Alteration in nutrition is related to depression. Decreased sexual activity is related to mood swings, depression, sleep disturbance, and fatigue. Figure 6-2 shows these associations and linkages.

As you study the complete (Fig. 6-3) web there are two areas where the arrows are concentrated: irregular exercise and decreased sexual activity. Using prototype identification and schema search, the health coach determined that focus on the irregular exercise would result in the most favorable outcomes in the shortest amount of time. Exercise and physical activity become the keystone issue. By focusing attention on the issue many of the other problems reported by Ms. White will be resolved.

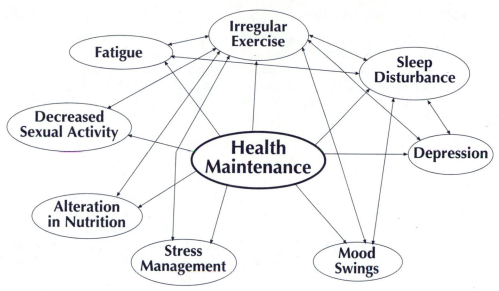

FIGURE 6-2 Developing Relationships in the Ms. Beth White Web

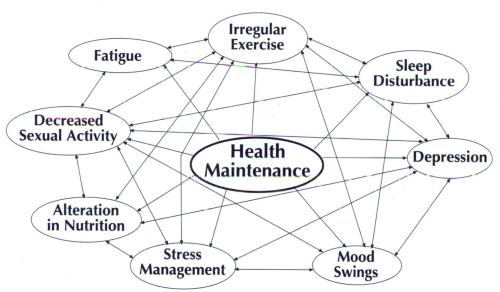

FIGURE 6-3 Clinical Reasoning Web for Ms. Beth White

Prototype Identification

Prototype identification involves use of a textbook case of wellness promotion as a reference point for comparative analysis. Ms. White's case represents one instance of the prototypical client of a professional woman with multiple life demands and a concern about maintaining her health and well-being. Knowing what the typical client with a health promotion challenge is likely to manifest serves as a standard for comparison and reasoning.

Schema Search

Schema search is the process of accessing general and/or specific patterns of past experiences that apply to the current situation. Past clinical experiences are helpful in reasoning about this specific case. For example, in this instance, the health coach has seen many women similar to Ms. White. The coach has a repertoire of experiences that help her understand and reason about what is most useful in this situation. The more experiences one gains, the greater the number of personal-history reference experiences one can bring to bear on present reasoning challenges. Given the fact pattern of Ms. White's story, do you have personal experiences that help you reason better and make sense of the facts? What experiences do you have that support your knowledge and understanding about the effects of exercise on mood and health?

Hypothesizing

Hypothesizing is determining an explanation that accounts for a set of facts that can be tested by further investigation. Given Ms. White's story, what set of facts needed explanations? Diagnostic hypotheses are guesses about what might explain her story. Diagnostic hypotheses are both the origins and insertion points as one creates a Clinical Reasoning Web. Hypothesizing involves if–then thinking. How are facts related? Hypothesis testing requires evidence. As one begins spinning and weaving the web it is easy to see how these diagnoses might be related through hypothesizing. If–then thinking supports and expands hypothesizing and influences thinking about the evidence needed to test hypotheses.

If–Then Thinking

If–then thinking involves logic and sequence of ideas and consequences. In Ms. White's case, what are some logical links and consequences? The nurse reasons that if sleep pattern disturbance is an issue then fatigue is a logical consequence. Sleep pattern disturbance could also influence mood. If activity and exercise were increased, then depression, sleep pattern disturbance, and mood could be positively influenced.

The nurse reflects and reasons. She knows that physical activity and exercise are key variable in the management of stress. An active exercise program is likely to influence the fatigue, sleep pattern disturbance, mood swings, poor coping skills, and depression. As she reflects and reasons about these relationships she draws connections on the web. She notices a convergence of arrows around the issue of exercise/physical activity. If exercise and physical activity is the keystone issue, then focusing on this as an area of intervention may have the most payoff in terms of health. For example, if Ms. White sustained an active exercise program, some of the other issues might be resolved?

Comparative Analysis

Identifying the keystone issue enables the nurse to focus care. Once a keystone issue is identified, it has a domino effect. Once Ms. White's activity and exercise regimen is activated it is likely to influence many of the other identified issues in the web. Comparative analysis is a thinking strategy that involves considering the strengths and weaknesses of competing alternatives. Once diagnostic hypotheses and their relationships are made explicit using the web, comparative analysis is used to determine which of these relationships is the keystone or the central supporting issues of Ms. White's case. Focusing care on the keystone issue is the most effective and efficient intervention choice.

STOP AND THINK

1. **What themes do you see in the Clinical Reasoning Web?**
2. **What present state does the theme suggest?**
3. **Given the present state, what outcome is suggested?**
4. **How does the simultaneous consideration of the themes, outcome state, and present state lead to framing the situation?**

One interpretation of the simultaneous consideration of Ms. White's story is the conclusion that health-seeking behaviors is a theme or frame for her situation. Once a frame has been identified, the stage is set for the concurrent consideration of where she is, where she wants to be, and what the gaps are in terms of her outcomes. Considering the present state of where she is with an outcome state of where she wants to be creates a test. The difference between these two states now becomes the focus of concern. What interventions or decisions need to be made to fill the gap? Based on the interventions or decisions, what is the evidence one needs to know the gap has been filled? Once one has evidence one needs to make judgments about what the evidence means given the context of the story, the frame and the clinical decisions the nurse makes. The following questions and thinking strategies help complete an OPT Model Worksheet.

STOP AND THINK

Outcome-Present State-Test (OPT)
1. **How does the frame influence the outcome state?**
2. **What evidence or criteria will indicate outcome achievement?**
3. **What influence does the frame have in creating the present state?**
4. **What test does the juxtaposition (side-by-side placement of the out-come state with present state) create?**
5. **What evidence is likely to be derived from this placement?**

Since health-seeking behavior is the frame or backdrop of Ms. White's story, an appropriate outcome based on reflection and analysis of the web is implementation of a regular exercise program. A minimum of three hours a week or 180 minutes of exercise is an identified outcome criteria. Using the thinking strategy of juxtaposition, one can contrast where Ms. White is (the present state of no structured exercise program) with where she needs/wants to be (a desired outcome state of 180 minutes of exercise per week). The gap between what is current and what is desirable needs to be filled with actions, decisions, and evidence. Juxtaposing helps create tests or the identification of the gaps between the current and desired states.

Juxtaposing

Juxtaposing involves putting the present state condition next to the outcome state. The side-by-side contrast of one state with the other illustrates the differences between the two states. The differences or gaps evident from the present to desired state help establish the conditions for the creation of a test in the OPT model. The gaps created give clues about the kind of evidence that is needed in order to make judgments regarding outcome achievement. Given Ms. White's case the nurse contrasts a decrease and alteration in physical activity with the desired outcome of a regular active exercise program of at least 180 minutes a week. The side-by-side comparison of these two states or conditions creates a test. There is a gap that must be bridged from one state to the other. In order to meet or match the desired outcome criteria of 180 minutes of exercise a week the nurse works with Ms. White to design an exercise program using the resources available to her. In Ms. White's case her firm subsidizes the services of personal trainers for their employees.

Given the frame of health-seeking behavior and the juxtaposing of present state and outcome state, a test between her present state of activity and a desired outcome state of 180 minutes per week is created. Will she meet the criteria of three hours of aerobic exercise a week? What other kinds of evidence will be derived from this gap analysis? What meaning will be attributed to the evidence? How will the evidence be helpful in making clinical judgments about outcome achievement?

STOP AND THINK

1. **What other test conditions can be created?**
2. **What is done to conduct the test and get evidence to fill the gap?**
3. **How are test results used to make clinical judgments?**
4. **What evidence is important in this case?**

To assist Ms. White in making the transition from the present state of decreased physical activity and exercise to the desired outcome of three hours of aerobic exercise a week, the nurse activated clinical decision making related to nursing actions and interventions to help her move from her present state to desired state. What specifically did the nurse do? How did she make choices about nursing actions useful to this situation? Active decision making influences reasoning.

Decision Making (Interventions)

Decision making involves making choices about nursing actions. The nursing intervention of exercise promotion seems to be the best choice to facilitate Ms. White's transition to her outcome state. Exercise promotion is one of the many nursing interventions classified in NIC. Remember, this knowledge classification system is a compilation of nursing interventions categorized by the Iowa Nursing Interventions Classification System project.

STOP AND THINK

1. **What nursing actions are necessary for outcome achievement?**
2. **How do nursing actions or clinical decisions promote achievement of the outcome state?**
3. **How do interventions relate to narrowing the gap between the present and desired states?**
4. **How do nursing interventions and decision making influence the creation of tests?**
5. **How do clinical decisions and nursing actions relate to the kind of evidence that is derived from the tests that are created?**
6. **What are the relationships between decision making and reflection?**

The nurse reflects, reasons, and decides that the nursing intervention of exercise promotion will have the most influence on the outcome. For example, Box 6-2 lists the nursing intervention activities associated with the intervention for exercise promotion.

BOX 6-2   Nursing Intervention Classification, Definition, and Activities for the Intervention of Exercise Promotion.

DEFINITION: Facilitation of regular physical exercise to maintain or advance to a higher level of fitness and health.

ACTIVITIES:

Appraise client's health beliefs regarding physical exercise.

Encourage verbalization of feelings regarding exercise or need for exercise.

Assist in identifying a positive role model for maintaining the exercise program.

Include client's family/caregivers in planning and maintaining the exercise program.

Inform client about health benefits and physiologic effects of exercise.

Instruct client about appropriate type of exercise for his or her level of health in collaboration with physician and/or exercise physiologist.

Instruct client about desired frequency, duration, and intensity of the exercise program.

Assist client to prepare and maintain a progress graph/chart to motivate adherence with the exercise program.

Instruct client about conditions warranting cessation of or alteration in the exercise program.

Instruct client on proper warm-up and cool-down exercises.

Instruct the client in techniques to avoid injury while exercising.

Instruct client in proper breathing techniques to maximize oxygen uptake during physical exercise.

Assist client to develop an appropriate exercise program to meet his or her needs.

Assist client to set short-term and long-term goals for the exercise program.

Assists client to schedule regular periods for the exercise program into weekly routine.

Provide reinforcement schedule to enhance client's motivation (e.g., weekly weigh-in).

Monitor client's response to exercise program.

Provide positive feedback for client's efforts.

Reprinted with permission from McCloskey, J. C., & Bulechek, G. M. (1996). *Nursing Intervention classification (2nd ed.).* St. Louis, MO: Mosby.

The nurse must continue to reflect, reason, and decide which of these interventions to use for Ms. White. The thinking strategies of comparative analysis and reflexive comparison help the nurse reason in this situation.

Reflexive Comparison

Reflexive comparison is a thinking strategy that involves constant comparison of the client's state from time of observation to time of observation. For example, next time Ms. White comes to see the nurse the results of her exercise efforts are reviewed. The nurse compares her progress from one observation or visit to the next. In this way the nurse is using both the identified outcome criteria and Ms. White as her own standard in terms of measuring progress toward the targeted exercise prescription. Based on these data the nurse conducts a test by juxtaposing the current or reported present state and outcome state data—has Ms. White achieved the outcome criteria of exercising 180 minutes per week? Clinical judgments are based on the evidence or meanings that are attributed to the results of the test. The simultaneous consideration of evidence, reflection, and decision making helps determine judgments.

There are three possible consequences of a test. First, Ms. White could achieve and match the desired outcome state of three hours of aerobic exercise activity per week. Second, her condition could deteriorate, necessitating simultaneous reflection, decision making, and perhaps reframing of the keystone issue. If the story changes the reasoning changes. Third, she could improve but not achieve the desired outcome. For example, she could achieve two hours of exercise. If this were the case then reflections about this are likely to provide new data and insights resulting in another set of clinical decisions or interventions to promote the transition to the outcome state. The consequences of these tests are the data one uses to make clinical judgments. Clinical judgments in the OPT model involve attributing meaning to the results of tests. Based on the evidence derived from the test, what does the evidence mean? Has the gap between present and desired states been narrowed or eliminated? Review the completed OPT Model Worksheet for Ms. White in Figure 6-4.

On her next visit Ms. White reports she has used the services of the firm's personal trainer. He comes to her house and brings an indoor rowing machine, exercise bike, weights, and stretch bands. Her trainer designed a program of aerobic activity and strength training for both Ms. White and her husband. The benefits of the exercise program are great. The trainer has challenged Ms. White and her husband to walk together early in the morning to provide them activity and time to talk with each other. Walking also contributes time toward the weekly exercise criteria of 180 minutes per week. The trainer spends 90 minutes a week with her and her husband. As a result of these sessions both Ms. White and her husband are losing weight, decreasing percentage body fat, and becoming more fit. Ms. White has experienced an increase in energy and feels more comfortable handling the stresses and strains at work.

After three months, Ms. White is feeling energized, active, and less stressed. She feels good about herself and enjoys the time that she and her husband spend walking and

OPT Model Worksheet

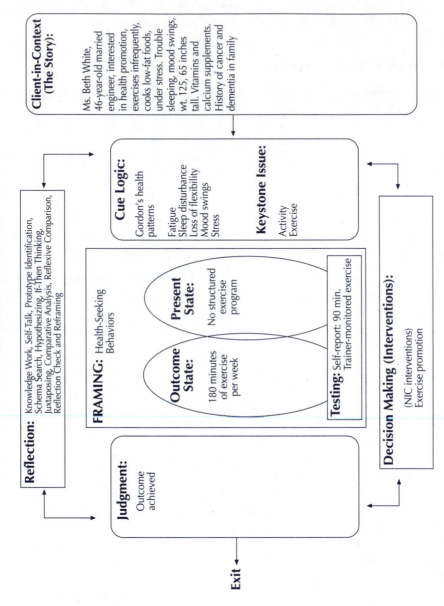

Reflection: Knowledge Work, Self-Talk, Prototype Identification, Schema Search, Hypothesizing, If-Then Thinking, Juxtaposing, Comparative Analysis, Reflexive Comparison, Reflection Check and Reframing

Client-in-Context (The Story):

Ms. Beth White, 46-year-old married engineer, interested in health promotion, exercises infrequently, cooks low-fat foods, under stress. Trouble sleeping, mood swings, wt. 125, 65 inches tall. Vitamins and calcium supplements. History of cancer and dementia in family

Cue Logic:

Gordon's health patterns

Fatigue
Sleep disturbance
Loss of flexibility
Mood swings
Stress

Keystone Issue:

Activity
Exercise

FRAMING: Health-Seeking Behaviors

Present State:

No structured exercise program

Outcome State:

180 minutes of exercise per week

Testing: Self-report: 90 min. Trainer-monitored exercise

Decision Making (Interventions):

(NIC interventions)
Exercise promotion

Judgment:

Outcome achieved

Exit

FIGURE 6-4 Completed OPT Model Worksheet for Ms. Beth White

exercising together. She is sleeping better, and is less depressed, and her moods seem to have stabilized. She is proud of the decrease in her body-mass index and percentage of body fat.

STOP AND THINK

1. **What evidence is important in this case?**
2. **What tests were created? What do the results of the tests mean?**
3. **What judgment can you make about outcome achievement?**
4. **How do judgments and reflections influence decision making?**
5. **How does experience with this case add to your clinical reasoning repertoire?**

Reframing

What if the results of Ms. White's tests were negative and she did not meet and achieve her desired outcome state criteria? Reasoning and reflection might lead to reframing. Reframing is the thinking strategy of attributing a different meaning to the facts. Once Ms. White reaches the outcome of achieving 180 minutes of exercise a week, the reasoning behind this issue is complete. If new issues emerged or were not resolved, then reflection and decision making would activate cue logic to frame other issues that emerge as prominent in the story. For example, what if Ms. White's stress, anxiety, and depression continue? If these states continued, then reflection and reasoning might result in reframing. Dialogue with her would likely lead to a different scenario. Working together the nurse and client would identify the most pressing present state and determine a desired outcome. Monitoring one's own thinking is a key skill. It is always helpful to self-evaluate one's thinking. A reflection check is good professional practice.

Reflection Check

Through use of a reflection check, one self-monitors, self-corrects, self-reinforces, and self-evaluates one's own thinking about a specific task or situation (Herman, Pesut, & Conard, 1994; Pesut & Herman, 1992; Worrell, 1990). A reflection check pinpoints what has been done correctly; it also identifies errors and provides insights and opportunities to identify and understand how to fix errors or reframe issues. The Stop and Think questions listed next might be helpful to Ms. White's nurse as she conducts a reflection check.

STOP AND THINK

1. Have I interpreted Ms. White's case correctly?
2. Am I satisfied with my analysis of ideas and arguments?
3. Have I made appropriate inferences, conjectures, and conclusions based on the evidence available?
4. Are my explanations sound in terms of logic, arguments, procedures, and results?
5. Are the claims and arguments for conducting and evaluating my tests sound?
6. How would an expert nurse perceive this situation?
7. What corrective measures, if any, do I need to take?

We presented Ms. White's story and illustrated use of the OPT model. As you review the story and the facts would you reason differently? With this case as an example, describe instances of your own use of self-talk, schema search, prototype identification, hypothesizing, if–then thinking, comparative analysis, juxtaposing, reflexive comparison, reframing, and reflection checking. Create your own Clinical Reasoning Web. Use the Thinking Strategies Worksheet in Table 6-2 to record your thoughts and answers.

STOP AND THINK

1. Explain how past clinical experiences influenced your reasoning about this case.
2. How will experience with this case influence future clinical reasoning given clients with a similar story?

SUMMARY

Maintaining and enhancing health is what primary care is all about. Healthy People 2000 identifies 21 priority areas for health promotion and disease prevention. Registered professional nurses are the health coaches of the future. Given the nation's emphasis on primary care, nurses who advocate health behavior and take their roles as health educators seriously are likely to be in great demand. The OPT model provides a structure for clinical reasoning in primary care contexts. Gordon's functional

TABLE 6-2 Thinking Strategies Worksheet		
THINKING STRATEGY	**DEFINITION**	**EXAMPLE FROM MS. WHITE**
Knowledge Work	Active use of reading, memorizing, drilling, writing, reviewing research, and practicing to learn clinical vocabulary	
Self-Talk	Expressing one's thoughts to one's self	
Schema Search	Accessing general and/or specific patterns of past experiences that might apply to the current situation	
Prototype Identification	Using a model case as a reference point for comparative analysis	
Hypothesizing	Determining an explanation that accounts for a set of facts that can be tested by further investigation	
If–Then Thinking	Linking ideas and consequences together in a logical sequence	
Comparative Analysis	Considering the strengths and weaknesses of competing alternatives	
Juxtaposing	Putting the present state condition next to the outcome state in a side-by-side contrast	
Reflexive Comparison	Constantly comparing the client's state from time of observation to time of observation	
Reframing	Attributing a different meaning to the content or context of a situation based on tests, decisions, or judgments	
Reflection Check	Self-examination and self-correction of critical thinking skills and thinking strategies that support clinical reasoning	

health pattern classification system enables nurses to quickly pinpoint health concerns in 11 functional areas. Gordon's functional health patterns provides a clinical vocabulary and content for clinical reasoning in primary care. According to Gordon, using the functional health patterns as an assessment guide enables one to quickly determine areas of strength and deviations from norms. The OPT model was used to structure reasoning about Ms. White's story. Application of the model was supported in terms of the reflective reasoning, critical thinking, and thinking strategies that make the model work. Since everyone reasons differently, readers were challenged at the end of the chapter to consider their reasoning about the case. The OPT model can be used in a primary health context to focus on wellness.

KEY CONCEPTS

1. Because of knowledge, skills, and abilities, nurses are ideal health coaches and educators.

2. Healthy People 2000 provides health promotion and disease prevention objectives for the nation.

3. Gordon's functional health patterns provides a useful way to assess primary health care needs and issues given client data and information.

4. The OPT model provides the structure for reasoning about well-being and health promotion. The model can be used in primary health care contexts.

5. The thinking strategies of self-talk, prototype identification, schema search, hypothesizing, if–then thinking, comparative analysis, reflexive comparison, reframing, and reflection check support the spinning and weaving of a Clinical Reasoning Web.

6. Reflection checks help develop critical thinking and reflective clinical reasoning.

STUDY QUESTIONS AND ACTIVITIES

1. Locate and read the latest report on the Health Status Objectives in your state given the Healthy People 2000 progress reports.

2. Based on data from your state, what health education, promotion, or disease prevention program can nurses create in order to achieve the health status objective identified in your locale? How can you use the OPT model to think about these program initiatives?

3. Conduct a health assessment on yourself. Use Gordon's functional health patterns and the OPT model to reason about your own wellness objectives. What would a Clinical Reasoning Web for you look like? How would you frame your issues and themes? What would your outcomes be? What are the gaps between where you are and where you want to be? What evidence would you use to test the narrowing of the gap?

4. NIC is an excellent resource for the clinical decisions nurses make. Find a copy of this resource and become familiar with its structure, organization, and contents.

REFERENCES

Bezold, C., & Mayer, E. (1996). *Future care: Responding to the demand for change.* New York: Faulkner & Gray.

Department of Health and Human Services. (1990). *Healthy People 2000: National health promotion and disease prevention objectives PHS 91-50212.* Washington, DC: US Government Printing Office.

Donaldson, M., Yordy, K., Lohr, K., and Vanselow, N. (Eds.). (1996). *Primary care: America's health in a new era.* Washington, DC: National Academy Press.

Dossey, B., Keegan, L., Guzzetta, C., & Kolkmeier, L. (1995). *Holistic nursing: A handbook for practice* (2nd ed.). Gaithersburg, MD: Aspen.

Herman, J. A., Pesut, D. J., & Conard, L. (1994). Using metacognitive skills: The quality audit. *Nursing Diagnosis, 5*(2), 56–64.

McCloskey, J. C., & Bulechek, G. M. (1996). *Nursing intervention classification* (2nd ed.). St. Louis, MO: Mosby.

North American Nursing Diagnosis Association. (1996). *Nursing diagnoses: Definitions and classifications, 1996–1998.* Philadelphia, PA: North American Nursing Diagnosis Association.

Pender, N. (1996). *Health promotion in nursing practice* (3rd ed.). Norwalk, CT: Appleton & Lange.

Pesut, D. J., & Herman, J. A. (1992). Metacognitive skills in diagnostic reasoning. *Nursing Diagnosis, 3*(4), 148–154.

Pesut, D. J., Herman, J. A., & Fowler, L. P. (1997). Toward a revolution in thinking: The OPT model of clinical reasoning. In J. McCloskey & H. Grace (Eds.), *Current issues in nursing* (5th ed., pp. 88–92). St. Louis, MO: Mosby.

Worrell, P. (1990). Metacognition: Implications for instruction in nursing education. *Journal of Nursing Education, 29,* 170–175.

CHAPTER 7

Clinical Reasoning in an Acute Care Context: The OPT Model and NANDA

COMPETENCIES

After completing this chapter, the reader should be able to:

1. Discuss the significance of acute care contexts in the continuum of care.

2. Identify selected issues in acute care contexts.

3. Apply the OPT model to an acute care case study.

4. Spin and weave a Clinical Reasoning Web given a case study.

5. Develop an OPT Model Worksheet for an acute care client.

6. Use the Thinking Strategies Worksheet to document examples of cue logic, framing, testing, reflection, clinical decision making, and clinical judgment in the case study scenario.

7. Practice reflection checks that support clinical reasoning.

8. Explain how reasoning and reflection influence thinking about clients in an acute care context.

INTRODUCTION

Although primary care is a health care goal, people do develop conditions that need attention in acute care treatment facilities. Acute care or hospital settings are contexts in which clinical reasoning takes place. The OPT model is useful for structuring thinking and reasoning in these settings. In this chapter, we discuss issues in acute care contexts. A postoperative knee replacement case is used as an example to support application of the OPT model. A Clinical Reasoning Web is created. The OPT Model Worksheet and Thinking Strategies Worksheets help guide reflection checks. A plan of care is created that relies on outcome specification, reflection, clinical decision making, and judgment. As you read and think about the case studies in this book, the OPT model will become more clear and understandable.

ACUTE CARE HEALTH CARE

The purpose of acute care is to provide an environment where health care professionals can implement intensive interventions, either medical or surgical, while constantly observing the outcomes of the treatment. These interventions are life-saving and life-sustaining. When individuals are too ill to care for themselves or to be treated in an outpatient setting, treatment in an inpatient setting is required. However, this type of care is expensive and separates individuals from their support systems. Therefore, one of the goals of acute care treatment is to manage the life-threatening or acute situation and return individuals to the community as quickly as possible.

Many of the diseases or illnesses that need attention in acute care contexts are identified in Healthy People 2000. People with heart disease, stroke, cancer, diabetes, chronic disabling disease, HIV, and infectious diseases are often treated at some time in an acute care setting. Acute care institutions provide environments where invasive diagnostic procedures, surgery, and emergency medical treatment can be performed.

In the United States the population is aging. Currently, 50 percent of all people admitted to an acute care institution are over the age of 75. This percentage will only increase and has consequences for the types of patients treated in acute care settings. The elderly suffer from more chronic illnesses, are sicker during an acute exacerbation, and recover slower. Because the prevailing practice is to keep people in the community, only the very sickest remain in an acute care institution. In fact, there is concern that acute care hospitals may become giant critical care units (Lemone & Burke, 1996).

NURSING KNOWLEDGE
IN ACUTE CARE: NANDA

The NANDA knowledge classification system was initiated in 1973. In the formative years, this classification system focused on client problems common in acute care settings. Initial nursing diagnoses were developed primarily by nurses working in these settings. It is an ideal classification system to use in the acute care context. Recall from an earlier chapter that NANDA categorizes patient states into one of nine human response patterns. Nursing diagnoses are clustered and organized around the concepts of: exchanging, communicating, relating, valuing, choosing, moving, perceiving, knowing, and feeling (NANDA, 1996). Each nursing diagnosis is accompanied by a list that includes a definition, defining characteristics, risk factors, and related factors. The definition is the description of the nursing diagnosis agreed upon by the membership of NANDA. The defining characteristics are the signs, symptoms, behaviors, and characteristics that a client displays when a specific nursing diagnosis is evident. Risk factors are the signs, symptoms, behaviors, characteristics, and environmental circumstances that put clients at risk for a specific nursing diagnosis. Related factors are the conditions or situations that influence the occurrence or maintenance of a nursing diagnosis (NANDA, 1996). Consider how nursing diagnoses from the NANDA classification system are used to reason about the case of Mr. George Smallwood.

CASE STUDY: MR. GEORGE SMALLWOOD'S STORY

George Smallwood is a divorced, 60-year-old white male Korean War Veteran. He is a recently retired construction worker who lives alone. He is the father of one child, a daughter, who is his reluctant primary caregiver. He presents to the Veterans Hospital complaining of severe pain in his right leg upon ambulating. After a complete medical assessment, Mr. Smallwood is found to be in good overall health but is diagnosed with degenerative joint disease of the right knee. He is scheduled for a knee replacement. This is his first hospital admission.

During right total knee replacement surgery, he lost approximately two pints of blood. He is prone to easy GI upset and states he has a "high tolerance for pain." He is eager to regain his independence and anxious to go home. At a glance, he seems like a "tough guy" who likes to be in control and not dependent on the health care team. Mr. Smallwood is in a significant amount of pain, which is evidenced by grimacing with movement of the right leg, yet he refuses to request oral pain medication. Overall, he has a positive disposition and is willing to apply a hard work ethic toward an aggressive rehabilitation. After his patient-controlled analgesia (PCA) pump was discontinued, he noted he was "experiencing good pain" on post-op day number two. He says that "pain makes me tired." Mr. Smallwood exhibits minor self-care deficits in bathing, grooming, and dressing; however, these deficiencies are normal for a second post-op day. His right knee is bandaged and braced. During the last dressing change, the surgical incision was healing appropriately without any signs or symptoms of redness, edema, or infection. Assessment of his leg reveals no signs of thrombophlebitis. His vital signs are stable.

STOP AND THINK

1. If you were Mr. Smallwood's nurse, how would you begin to reason about his care?
2. How might the OPT model assist you in structuring your reflections and reasoning?
3. What cues are associated with his story?
4. How would you develop the cue logic associated with Mr. Smallwood's story?
5. How would you arrange the points and diagnostic possibilities on a Clinical Reasoning Web?
6. What are your initial thoughts about the frame for this situation?
7. What outcome is desirable?

SPINNING AND WEAVING THE CLINICAL REASONING WEB

As the nurse listened to Mr. Smallwood she made mental notes using the NANDA patterns as a guide. Listed in Table 7-1 are the human response patterns, supporting data, and diagnostic hypotheses she recorded for each NANDA pattern.

THINKING STRATEGIES THAT SUPPORT REFLECTIVE CLINICAL REASONING

It is difficult to generate diagnostic hypotheses for Mr. Smallwood's case study without the prerequisite knowledge work. For example, if one did not know the definitions, classifications, and categories of diagnoses associated with NANDA it would be difficult to pinpoint issues, concerns, deviations, or areas that might benefit from intervention. Other foundation knowledge needed to plan care for Mr. Smallwood includes knowledge about physiological, psychological, and sociological responses to surgery. Knowledge in these areas include facts about normal postoperative trajectory, complications following surgery, and individual variations in people's pain-coping strategies. Knowledge in these areas helps one to interpret, analyze, and explain some of the issues surrounding reasoning and planning care for Mr. Smallwood. Reasoning is supported by the reflection strategies of self-talk, schema search, prototype identification, hypothesizing, and if–then thinking. Consider how these apply to the development of the Clinical Reasoning Web for Mr. Smallwood.

TABLE 7-1 Human Response Patterns, Data, and Hypotheses from Mr. George Smallwood's Story

HUMAN RESPONSE PATTERN	DATA	DIAGNOSTIC HYPOTHESES
Pattern 1: Exchanging	Lost two units of blood during surgery Surgical incision Surgery impairs normal mode of transport	Fluid volume deficit Risk for injury Risk for infection
Pattern 2: Communicating	No data	
Pattern 3: Relating	No data	
Pattern 4: Valuing	No data	
Pattern 5: Choosing	No data	
Pattern 6: Moving	Leg is braced and elevated Unable to walk at present, but will begin physical therapy soon Unable to get up and go to bathroom Surgery creates minor problems in bathing, grooming, and dressing "Pain makes me tired"	Impaired physical mobility Activity intolerance Self-care deficit—toileting Fatigue
Pattern 7: Perceiving	Knee replaced with artificial joint	Body image disturbance
Pattern 8: Knowing	First hospital admission Does not know what is going to happen in rehabilitation Interested in learning how to be independent	Knowledge deficit
Pattern 9: Feeling	Grimacing when leg is moved Refuses oral pain meds "Experiencing good pain" Anxious to go home Anxiety about dependency	Acute pain Anxiety

Self-Talk

"What are the nursing diagnostic possibilities for postoperative care associated with knee replacement surgery?" Self-talk is the process of expressing one's thoughts to oneself. Self-talk enables you to pose questions. The answer to these questions results in the identification of the diagnostic hypotheses relevant to the case. In this instance the nurse decided to use the NANDA human response patterns as the knowledge classification system to guide thinking and reasoning. Each human response pattern was identified. Through the use of self-talk the nurse then asked or posed the question, "Given the story, what possible nursing diagnoses are associated with each of the nine human response patterns?" Answers to this question reveal such possibilities as fluid volume deficit, risk for infection, risk for injury, knowledge deficit, impaired physical mobility, activity intolerance, fatigue, body image disturbance, self-care deficit, acute pain, and anxiety. The web is begun by placing total knee replacement in the center and then adding all the nursing diagnostic possibilities around the outer edges. Consider the beginning Clinical Reasoning Web that was developed for Mr. Smallwood. (See Figure 7-1.)

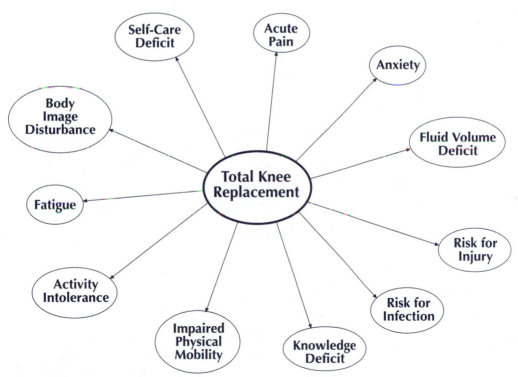

FIGURE 7-1 Beginning the Clinical Reasoning Web for Mr. George Smallwood

These diagnoses become the basis for care planning. The diagnoses were derived from Mr. Smallwood's story. The diagnoses are the nursing-focused consequences of his surgical treatment and condition.

Prototype Identification

Mr. Smallwood's case represents one instance of the prototypical postoperative client. Knowing what the typical client with a postoperative knee replacement trajectory experiences enables one to better compare Mr. Smallwood's progress with the prototype. Prototype identification is using a model case as a reference point for comparative analysis. Prototypes serve as one standard of care to use as a reference point for comparative analysis. Nursing care issues for postoperative clients involve attention to respiratory status, pain control, wound care, ambulation, prevention of infection, fluid replacement, rehabilitation, and surveillance for potential complications. All of this information is derived from reading and studying reference materials and current nursing research literature, and applying knowledge of the prototype to the specific case of Mr. Smallwood. Knowledge work enhances prototype understanding.

Schema Search

Past clinical experiences are helpful in reasoning about specific cases. The nurse may or may not have experience working with clients similar to Mr. Smallwood. Schema search is the process of accessing general and/or specific patterns of past experiences that might apply to the current situation. Remembering past experiences supports and enhances the reasoning process. Think of past clinical experiences that might help you understand and make the connections and linkages given Mr. Smallwood's case.

Hypothesizing

When spinning and weaving the Clinical Reasoning Web, one has to think out loud and reason about the possible relationships and connections among these diagnostic hypotheses. Hypothesizing is determining an explanation that accounts for a set of facts that can be tested by further investigation. Hypothesizing presupposes the use and understanding of clinical vocabulary. For example, during self-talk cues lead to diagnoses. Diagnoses are matched with cues. Preliminary thoughts about diagnostic hypotheses emerge. Hypotheses are guesses about what might explain some of the nursing care issues in Mr. Smallwood's story.

Diagnostic hypotheses become both origins and insertion points in a Clinical Reasoning Web. Each diagnosis could be the focus of care. However, as one considers associations among the possibilities a keystone issue is likely to emerge that will serve to organize the focus of care and influence other nursing care concerns. The number of nursing diagnoses associated with clients who need postoperative care is great. Therefore, it becomes important to identify the keystone issue or issues requiring intervention. The identification and description of relationships between and among the diagnostic hypotheses enables the nurse to determine crucial issues that focus nursing care planning. If–then thinking supports identification of the keystone issue.

If–Then Thinking

If–then thinking involves linking ideas and consequences together in a logical sequence. In Mr. Smallwood's case, here are some possible linkages that can be made. The nurse reasons that there is a relationship between pain and mobility, pain and self-care and several other diagnostic hypotheses in the web. For example, there are relationships between risk for injury, knowledge deficit, self-care deficit, and impaired physical mobility. Fatigue can be related to anxiety, self-care deficit, fluid volume deficit, and activity intolerance. Impaired physical mobility can be related to body image disturbance, anxiety, risk for injury, and self-care deficit. Look at Figure 7-2 and note how the relationships are represented on the web. What other diagnostic hypotheses are obviously related?

Analyze the web. Note the convergence of functional relationships around a keystone issue. Consider the links and relationships between impaired mobility and pain. Doesn't it make sense that if Mr. Smallwood managed his pain, his mobility would increase and many of the other issues identified would resolve? Figure 7-3 contains a completed web for Mr. Smallwood.

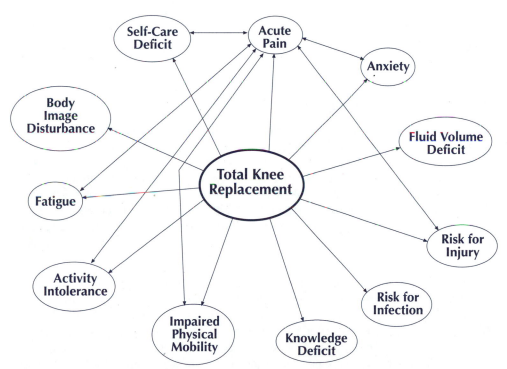

FIGURE 7-2 Developing Relationships in the Mr. George Smallwood Web

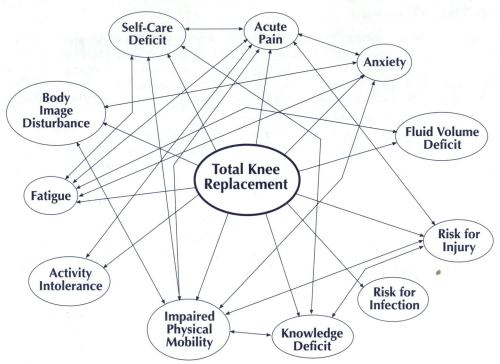

FIGURE 7-3   Clinical Reasoning Web for Mr. George Smallwood

Comparative Analysis

Once diagnostic hypotheses and their relationships are made explicit using the web, comparative analysis is used to determine which of these relationships is the keystone or central supporting issues of Mr. Smallwood's case. Identifying the keystone issue enables the nurse to focus care. Once a keystone issue is identified, it has a domino effect. Once we take care of Mr. Smallwood's pain and impaired physical mobility, this is likely to influence the other identified issues such as self-care deficit, anxiety, fatigue, body image disturbance, and risk for injury. Comparative analysis is a thinking strategy that involves considering the strengths and weaknesses of competing alternatives.

Concurrent consideration of client-in-context and the Clinical Reasoning Web leads to the conclusion that postoperative care is an organizing theme or frame for Mr. Smallwood's case. In many postoperative situations, problems with mobility and pain management lead to other problems, such as pneumonia, wound infection, constipation, paralytic ileus, and pressure ulcers. Nursing interventions addressing the keystone issues in this case are organized around postoperative nursing care concerns.

STOP AND THINK

1. **What themes do you see in the Clinical Reasoning Web?**
2. **What do you think is most important? Why is your observation the most important?**
3. **Given the present state, what outcome is suggested?**
4. **How does simultaneous consideration of the outcome state, present state, and frame lead to specification of test and the type of evidence needed to satisfy the test?**
5. **How does past experience and knowledge of postoperative care needs influence your thinking and clinical decision making regarding choice of nursing actions?**

Once a frame has been identified, the stage is set for consideration of present state, outcome state, and test. Look at the completed OPT Model Worksheet (Figure 7-4). Since the frame for thinking about Mr. Smallwood's situation is postoperative care, what outcome state and present state juxtaposition does this suggest, and how can a test be created and established?

STOP AND THINK

1. **What influence does the frame have on the outcome state?**
2. **What evidence will indicate outcome achievement?**
3. **How does the frame influence identification of the present state?**
4. **What test does the juxtaposition or contrast of outcome state with present state create?**
5. **What difference can be determined by this side-by-side comparison?**
6. **What evidence can be derived from this test?**

Given postoperative care as the frame for Mr. Smallwood's story, an appropriate outcome based on reflection and analysis of the web is achievement of mobility and comfort. Juxtaposing or side-by-side comparison helps support the reasoning process.

OPT Model Worksheet

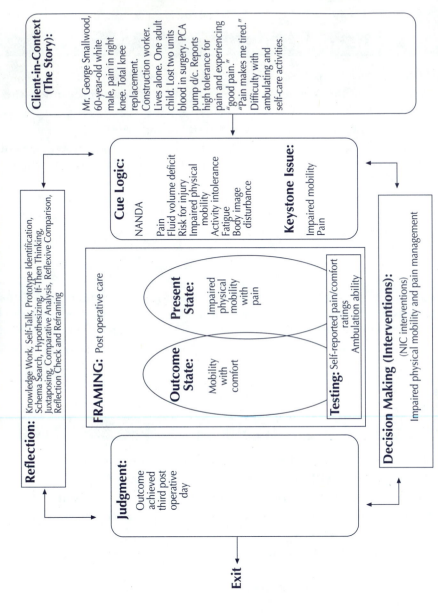

Reflection: Knowledge Work, Self-Talk, Prototype Identification, Schema Search, Hypothesizing, If-Then Thinking, Juxtaposing, Comparative Analysis, Reflexive Comparison, Reflection Check and Reframing

Client-in-Context (The Story):

Mr. George Smallwood, 60-year-old white male, pain in right knee. Total knee replacement. Construction worker. Lives alone. One adult child. Lost two units blood in surgery. PCA pump d/c. Reports high tolerance for pain and experiencing "good pain." "Pain makes me tired." Difficulty with ambulating and self-care activities.

Cue Logic:

NANDA

Pain
Fluid volume deficit
Risk for injury
Impaired physical mobility
Activity intolerance
Fatigue
Body image disturbance

Keystone Issue:

Impaired mobility
Pain

FRAMING: Post operative care

Present State:

Impaired physical mobility with pain

Outcome State:

Mobility with comfort

Testing: Self-reported pain/comfort ratings
Ambulation ability

Decision Making (Interventions):

(NIC interventions)
Impaired physical mobility and pain management

Judgment:

Outcome achieved third post operative day

Exit

FIGURE 7-4 Completed OPT Model Worksheet for Mr. George Smallwood

Juxtaposing

Juxtaposing involves putting the present state condition next to the outcome state. The side-by-side contrast of one state with the other illustrates the differences between the two states. The differences or gaps evident from the contrast of present to desired state help establish the conditions for a test in the OPT model. From this test evidence is derived. Evidence derived supports judgment and reflection.

In Mr. Smallwood's case the nurse contrasts impaired mobility with the desired outcome of mobility with comfort. The side-by-side comparison of these two states or conditions creates a test. There is a gap that must be bridged from one state to the other. In order to meet or match the desired outcome criteria of mobility with comfort the nurse will need to make clinical decisions and choose nursing actions and interventions to bridge the gap. Decisions that one makes and interventions one initiates help bridge the gap between juxtaposed conditions.

A test is developed concurrently with the juxtaposition and decisions about the outcome state. Given the frame of postoperative nursing care and the juxtaposing of present state and outcome state, a test between Mr. Smallwood's present state of impaired mobility with pain and a desired outcome state for mobility with comfort is created.

STOP AND THINK

1. **What other test conditions can be created?**
2. **What evidence can be derived from these test conditions?**
3. **How is the evidence or test results used to make clinical judgments?**
4. **How does past experience influence reflection and action?**

To assist Mr. Smallwood in the transition from the present state of impaired mobility with pain to the desired outcome of mobility with comfort, the nurse activated clinical decision making related to nursing actions and interventions that help him make the transition from his state of immobility with pain to one of mobility with comfort. The nurse uses knowledge contained in NIC's intervention categories to make clinical decisions about nursing actions.

Decision Making (Interventions)

NIC is a knowledge classification system that provides guidance concerning activities and nursing interventions. The nurse must decide among an array of possible interventions. For example, Box 7-1 identifies nursing interventions that could be used to assist Mr. Smallwood with management of mobility.

BOX 7-1 Nursing Intervention Classification, Definition, and Activities for the Intervention for Physical Mobility

DEFINITION: A state in which an individual experiences a limitation of ability for independent physical movement

SUGGESTED NURSING INTERVENTIONS FOR PROBLEM RESOLUTION:

Bed Rest Care
Cerebral Perfusion Promotion
Energy Management
Environmental Management
Exercise Promotion
Exercise Promotion: Stretching
Exercise Therapy: Ambulation
Exercise Therapy: Balance
Exercise Therapy: Joint Mobility

Exercise Therapy: Muscle Control
Positioning
Positioning: Intraoperative
Positioning: Neurologic
Positioning: Wheelchair
Self-Care Assistance
Teaching: Prescribed Activity/Exercise
Traction/Immobilization Care

ADDITIONAL OPTIONAL INTERVENTIONS:

Activity Therapy
Autogenic Training
Body Mechanics Promotion
Biofeedback
Cast Care: Maintenance
Cast Care: Wet
Circulatory Care
Circulatory Precautions
Distraction
Fall Prevention
Foot Care
Hypnosis
Labor Suppression
Medication Management
Meditation

Neurologic Monitoring
Pain Management
Pass Facilitation
Peripheral Sensation Management
Phototherapy: Neonate
Physical Restraint
Pressure Management
Progressive Muscle Relaxation
Prosthesis Care
Simple Massage
Surveillance: Safety
Skin Surveillance
Splinting
Therapeutic Touch
Weight Management

Reprinted with permission from McCloskey, J. C., & Bulechek, G. M. (1996). *Nursing intervention classification* (2nd ed.). St. Louis, MO: Mosby.

Clinical decisions are needed to make choices about the pain management techniques that will be most helpful for Mr. Smallwood. Box 7-2 lists the interventions and choices the nurse will consider in working toward increasing his comfort and decreasing his pain.

Other clinical decisions the nurse needs to make are related to teaching prescribed activity/exercise or self-care assistance techniques. The nurse must also decide about the degree of clinical surveillance needed around the issues of safety and skin integrity. Linking interventions with diagnoses comes with experience. However, a

---

BOX 7-2   Nursing Intervention Classification, Definition, and Activities for Intervention for Pain

DEFINITION: A state in which an individual experiences and reports the presence of severe discomfort or an uncomfortable sensation.

SUGGESTED NURSING INTERVENTIONS FOR PROBLEM RESOLUTION:

Acupressure

Analgesic Administration

Analgesic Administration: Intraspinal

Anesthesia Administration

Anxiety Reduction

Conscious Sedation

Cutaneous Stimulation

Environmental Management: Comfort

Flatulence Reduction

Medication Administration

Medication Administration: Interpleural

Medication Management

Medication Prescribing

Pain Management

Patient-Controlled Analgesia (PCA)

Rectal Prolapse Management

Transcutaneous Electrical Nerve
  Stimulation (TENS)

ADDITIONAL OPTIONAL INTERVENTIONS:

Animal-Assisted Therapy

Autogenic Training

Bathing

Biofeedback

Bowel Management

Coping Enhancement

Distraction

Energy Management

Environmental Management

Exercise Promotion

Exercise Promotion: Stretching

Exercise Therapy: Balance

Exercise Therapy: Joint Mobility

Exercise Therapy: Muscle Control

Hope Installation

Humor

Hypnosis

Meditation

Music Therapy

Oxygen Therapy

Positioning

Preparatory Sensory Information

Presence

Progressive Muscle Relaxation

Security Enhancement

Simple Guided Imagery

Simple Massage

Simple Relaxation Therapy

Sleep Enhancement

Therapeutic Touch

Touch

Vital Signs Monitoring

Reprinted with permission from McCloskey, J. C., & Bulechek, G. M. (1996). *Nursing intervention classification* (2nd ed.). St. Louis, MO: Mosby.

---

resource that does some linking of nursing interventions and nursing diagnoses can be found in Part IV of the NIC text authored by McCloskey and Bulechek (1996).

How is the nurse going to assist Mr. Smallwood in moving from a state of impaired mobility with pain to the state of mobility with comfort? The goal of this decision making is to select the interventions and actions that will have the most influence on the outcome. Following application of the interventions, the nurse will evaluate progress of outcome achievement. Through the use of the thinking strategy of reflexive

STOP AND THINK

1. **Given the reflective reasoning involved with Mr. Smallwood's story, what nursing actions are necessary for outcome achievement?**
2. **How will the choice of nursing actions or clinical decisions promote achievement of outcome state?**
3. **Which nursing interventions are most useful to achieve the outcome?**
4. **Which nursing interventions are not a good choice given the facts of the story?**

comparison, the nurse will use Mr. Smallwood as his own standard of measurement of outcome achievement.

Reflexive Comparison

Reflexive comparison involves constant comparison of the client's state from time of observation to time of observation. For example, the nurse will compare Mr. Smallwood's progress with mobility and comfort from one day to the next until discharge. In this way the nurse is using both the identified outcome criteria and Mr. Smallwood as his own standard in terms of making progress toward the desired outcome state. Based on this data, the nurse will gather evidence from side-by-side tests or by juxtaposing frequent comparisons of present state—where Mr. Smallwood is with where he would like to be given the outcome state criteria. Evidence gathered supports three possible consequences. First, Mr. Smallwood could achieve and match the desired outcome state of mobility with comfort. Second, his condition could deteriorate. The story could change, requiring reflection and action. Third, Mr. Smallwood might make progress but not achieve or meet the desired outcome. Based on evidence derived from tests, one would reflect and make judgments.

Clinical judgments are the meanings that are attributed to evidence derived from test results based on reflexive comparisons. The concurrent consideration of reflexive comparisons, test results, judgment, reflection, and decision making determines the continued need for clinical reasoning. For example, what clinical judgment would you make if you were given the following facts? On the third postoperative day, Mr. Smallwood is able to transfer from the bed to a wheelchair with no grimacing and no verbal report of any pain. He has begun a physical therapy routine and has achieved increased range of motion in his joint and is beginning to use crutches.

Since the outcome state was achieved, the nurse turned her attention toward Mr. Smallwood's discharge planning. Given the frame of discharge planning, home maintenance and health management become the focus of reflective clinical reasoning, outcome specification, and clinical decision making. The concurrent nature of clinical reasoning continues as Mr. Smallwood anticipates discharge.

STOP AND THINK

1. **What evidence is derived from the test?**
2. **How do the evidence and reflexive comparison influence judgment?**
3. **How do reflection and judgment influence clinical decision making?**
4. **How does the simultaneous consideration of judgment, reflection, and decision making influence reframing and the development of Mr. Smallwood's story?**

Reframing

Suppose clinical judgments associated with the reasoning about Mr. Smallwood's case were not positive and he did not achieve mobility with comfort. The facts of the story then change and require a different explanation. When the meaning of the set of facts changes, reframing the situation is necessary. Reframing is a thinking strategy that involves attributing a different meaning to the content or context of a situation given a set of facts or judgments. How might you attribute a different meaning to the facts of Mr. Smallwood's case? Suppose a colleague used the frame of fatigue and energy management rather than post-op care as the initial framing?

STOP AND THINK

1. **Was Mr. Smallwood's case interpreted correctly?**
2. **If not, how would you organize elements of the story using the OPT model structure?**

Reflection Check

A reflection check pinpoints what has been done correctly; it also identifies errors and provides insights and opportunities to identify and understand how to fix errors or reframe issues. Explain how experience with this case will influence future clinical reasoning given clients with a similar story. Review the case and use the Thinking Strategies Worksheet in Table 7-2 to identify examples of each of the thinking strategies.

TABLE 7-2 Thinking Strategies Worksheet

THINKING STRATEGY	DEFINITION	EXAMPLE FROM GEORGE SMALLWOOD'S CASE
Knowledge Work	Active use of reading, memorizing, drilling, writing, reviewing research, and practicing to learn clinical vocabulary	
Self-Talk	Expressing one's thoughts to one's self	
Schema Search	Accessing general and/or specific patterns of past experiences that might apply to the current situation	
Prototype Identification	Using a model case as a reference point for comparative analysis	
Hypothesizing	Determining an explanation that accounts for a set of facts that can be tested by further investigation	
If–Then Thinking	Linking ideas and consequences together in a logical sequence	
Comparative Analysis	Considering the strengths and weaknesses of competing alternatives	
Juxtaposing	Putting the present-state condition next to the outcome state in a side by-side contrast	
Reflexive Comparison	Constantly comparing the client's state from time of observation to time of observation	
Reframing	Attributing a different meaning to the content or context of a situation based on tests, decisions, or judgments	
Reflection Check	Self-examination and self-correction of critical thinking skills and thinking strategies that support clinical reasoning	

SUMMARY

In this chapter we discussed clinical reasoning in an acute care context. We illustrated use of the OPT model with diagnoses most often associated with postoperative clients. We analyzed and reasoned through the story of Mr. Smallwood, a 60-year-old man who received a total knee replacement. Using the clinical vocabulary of NANDA and NIC, we applied the Clinical Reasoning Web and OPT Model Worksheet and discussed the thinking strategies that support clinical reasoning. In the next chapter we discuss use of the OPT model and the Omaha classification system for structuring reasoning in the context of community nursing.

KEY CONCEPTS

1. The purpose of acute care is to provide an environment where health care professionals can implement intensive interventions. These interventions are life-saving and life-sustaining.

2. Acute care is expensive and separates individuals from their support systems. Therefore, the goal of acute care is to manage the life-threatening or acute situation and return individuals to the community as quickly as possible.

3. Clinical reasoning in acute care contexts is facilitated by use of the OPT model.

4. The NANDA classification system focuses on client problems common in acute care settings and was developed primarily by nurses working in these settings. It is an ideal classification system to use in the acute care context.

5. Nursing care issues for postoperative clients involve attention to respiratory status, pain control, wound care, ambulation, prevention of infection, fluid replacement, rehabilitation, and surveillance for potential complications. All of this information is derived from the knowledge work of reading and studying reference materials and current nursing research literature, and applying knowledge of the prototype to the specific case of Mr. Smallwood.

6. The thinking strategies of self-talk, schema search, prototype identification, hypothesizing, and if–then thinking support creation of a Clinical Reasoning Web.

7. NIC organizes nursing interventions from which nurses make clinical decisions and choices concerning activities and interventions that help clients make the transition from present states to desired outcomes states.

8. Each reasoning experience with clients in acute care contexts adds to one's professional history and provides reference experiences for future clinical reasoning challenges.

STUDY QUESTIONS AND ACTIVITIES

1. Identify an acute care facility in your community. Find out the most frequently performed surgical interventions. Based on this information,

what nursing diagnoses can you predict are the most prevalent in that setting?

2. Interview a nurse who practices in an acute care setting. Ask her to share her observations about the most critical nursing care needs of clients in this setting.

3. While the focus of this chapter was on the surgical patient, some clients in these facilities are hospitalized for medical management. For example, an elderly person with diabetes might spend time in an acute care facility. How might your thinking, reasoning, and care planning be different or the same for this client?

4. Imagine you had the knee replacement that Mr. Smallwood experienced in the scenario described in this chapter. What nursing care actions and interventions would be most important to your recovery? What would you expect in terms of nursing care?

REFERENCES

Department of Health and Human Services. (1990). *Healthy People 2000: National heath promotion and disease prevention objectives* PHS 91-50212. Washington, DC: US Government Printing Office.

Lemone, P., & Burke, K. (1996). *Medical surgical nursing: Critical thinking in client care.* Menlo Park, CA: Addison-Wesley.

McCloskey, J., & Bulechek, G. (1996). *Nursing intervention classification* (2nd ed.). St. Louis, MO: Mosby.

North American Nursing Diagnosis Association. (1996). *Nursing diagnoses: Definitions and classifications 1997–1998*. Philadelphia, PA: North American Nursing Diagnosis Association.

CHAPTER 8

Clinical Reasoning in Community Care: Using the OPT Model and the Omaha Nursing Classification System

COMPETENCIES

After completing this chapter, the reader should be able to:

1. Use the OPT model and the Omaha nursing classification system for structuring the reasoning and case study content given a community health context.

2. Explain how the OPT model and the diagnosis, intervention, and outcome rating scheme of the Omaha classification system support clinical reasoning in community contexts.

3. Spin and weave a Clinical Reasoning Web using information about a client who is blind, diabetic, and homebound.

4. Develop an OPT Model Worksheet for a client who requires care in the community.

5. Explain the clinical reasoning and thinking strategies associated with reasoning about the case study.

6. Analyze the usefulness of the Omaha classification system as a knowledge classification system that supports reasoning in community health contexts.

INTRODUCTION

In this chapter, the Omaha nursing classification system is used to support reasoning about a client needing care in the home. As you work through this example, compare and contrast the diagnosis, intervention, and problem-rating scheme of the Omaha nursing classification system with the other nursing knowledge systems discussed earlier in this text. After reading the chapter and studying the case example, consider the advantages and disadvantages of the Omaha nursing classification system. Make a judgment about the system's usefulness for reasoning about client care needs in the community.

COMMUNITY CARE AND CLINICAL REASONING

Health care is moving from hospitals into communities. Community care is a venue for practice that allows autonomy for the nurse. In a community context nursing values support client values for disease prevention, health promotion and maintenance, or recovery from illness. Some authors argue that theory-based practice in the community is the crux of professional nursing (Clarke & Cody, 1994). In the community, clinicians learn from clients who maintain health in the context of their homes. Community health nurses appreciate how systems interact in order to achieve health outcomes. Community care often focuses on issues related to environmental health. Community care also highlights psychosocial, physiological, and health-behavior related issues. Categories of interventions in the community consist of health teaching, guidance and counseling, and disease prevention. Interventions include administration of treatments and procedures, case management, and surveillance. In some cases, care planning and resource acquisition for clients and communities require political action. When thinking and reasoning in a community context, one needs to consider how clients fit into the big picture of public policy, resource allocation, and health programming efforts. The Omaha nursing classification system has been developed over the past 20 years specifically for community contexts.

ORGANIZED NURSING KNOWLEDGE FOR COMMUNITY CARE: THE OMAHA CLASSIFICATION SYSTEM

The Omaha classification system is an example of a practice-based effort to name activities involved in nursing practice (Martin & Scheet, 1995). The Omaha Community Health System (OCHS) consists of standardized terms for nursing diagnoses, interventions, and ratings of problems and outcomes. The problem classification scheme consists of over 40 client problems organized around four areas of concern: the environment, psychosocial issues, physiological issues, and health-related behaviors. Definitions of each area and examples of client problems within each domain are listed in Box 8-1.

BOX 8-1   Domain and Problem Categories of the Omaha Nursing Classification System

Domain I. Environmental: The material resources, physical surroundings, and substances both internal and external to client, home, neighborhood, and broader community

- **01.** Income
- **02.** Sanitation
- **03.** Residence
- **04.** Neighborhood/workplace safety
- **05.** Other

Domain II. Psychosocial: Patterns of behavior, communication, relationship, and development

- **06.** Communication with community resources
- **07.** Social contact
- **08.** Role change
- **09.** Interpersonal relationship
- **10.** Spiritual distress
- **11.** Grief
- **12.** Emotional stability
- **13.** Human sexuality
- **14.** Caretaking/parenting
- **15.** Neglected child/adult
- **16.** Abused child/adult
- **17.** Growth and development
- **18.** Other

Domain III. Physiological: Functional status of processes that maintain life

- **19.** Hearing
- **20.** Vision
- **21.** Speech and language
- **22.** Dentition
- **23.** Cognition
- **24.** Pain
- **25.** Consciousness
- **26.** Integument
- **27.** Neuromusculoskeletal function
- **28.** Respiration
- **29.** Circulation
- **30.** Digestion-hydration
- **31.** Bowel function
- **32.** Genitourinary function
- **33.** Antepartum/postpartum
- **34.** Other

continued

Domain IV. Health-Related Behaviors: Activities that maintain or promote wellness, promote recovery, or maximize rehabilitation potential

35. Nutrition
36. Sleep and rest patterns
37. Physical activity
38. Personal hygiene
39. Substance use
40. Family planning
41. Health care supervision
42. Prescribed medication regimen
43. Technical procedure
44. Other

Reprinted with permission from Norma M. Lang, PhD, RN, FAAN, FRCN, editor, *Nursing Data Systems: The Emerging Framework* © 1995 American Nurses Publishing, American Nurses Foundation/American Nurses Association, 600 Maryland Avenue, SW, Suite 100W, Washington, DC 20024-2571.

Approximately 44 nursing diagnoses are listed in the four areas and represent many of the problems within the scope of community health nursing practice. One of the unique aspects of OCHS is the attempt to relate problems with interventions and outcomes. Outcomes in this knowledge system are defined as changes in knowledge, behavior, and status of a given problem. An outcome problem-rating scale helps one judge if outcomes have been achieved. Parts of the Omaha system are described in the following sections.

Problem Domains

The Omaha system supports a problem identification approach to nursing care. Client problems are organized in four areas called domains: environmental, psychosocial, physiological, and health-related behaviors. The domains and examples of problems in each category are described in the next four paragraphs.

The environmental domain consists of concerns about physical surroundings, including the home, the neighborhood, and the community in which the client resides. Material and natural resources are also considered part of the environmental domain. Examples of problems in the environmental domain relate to financial, sanitation, residential, and safety issues.

The psychosocial domain involves behavioral patterns, communication issues, relationships, and issues of growth and development. Examples of problems in the psychosocial domain are communication exchanges with community resources, social contact, role changes, interpersonal relationships, spiritual distress, grief, emotional stability, and human sexuality. Other issues such as caretaking, parenting, neglect, child abuse, grief, and spiritual distress are classified under this category.

The physiological domain is defined by those processes that maintain life. Problems classified in this area include difficulties with hearing, vision, speech and language, dentition, cognition, and pain. Nursing care problems associated with consciousness, integumentary, neuromusculoskeletal function, respiration, circulation, digestion, bowel/bladder functions, antepartum/postpartum, and "other" issues are included in this domain. For example, a specific problem associated with circulation like "irregular heart rate" would be included in this domain.

The fourth and final problem area of the Omaha system is defined in terms of health-related behaviors. In this problem domain are behaviors and activities that maintain or promote wellness, aid in recovery, or maximize rehabilitation. For example, problems listed in this domain relate to nutrition, sleep and rest patterns, physical activity, personal hygiene, substance use, family planning, and health care supervision. Specific problems in this domain include issues such as "sedentary lifestyle" under the problem of physical activity and "abuses alcohol" under the problem of substance use.

Modifiers are used to specify and qualify the problems. (Refer to Box 8-1.) Modifiers include individual, family, health promotion, potential, deficit, or actual impairment. For example, under the domain of health-related behaviors, a problem may be substance use and the specific problem is "smoking." If a client does not smoke but someone around him does and encourages the client to participate, the modifier would be "potential" for smoking.

STOP AND THINK

1. **To what degree do you think the problems in the Omaha nursing classification system capture the scope of nursing care problems in community health contexts?**
2. **Compare and contrast the 44 problems identified in the Omaha system with the 11 functional health patterns of Gordon.**
3. **How are the Omaha problems similar to and different from NANDA diagnoses?**
4. **To what degree is nursing practice in a community health context different from that in an acute care context?**
5. **Do you believe practice in a community health context is different enough to warrant a unique nursing knowledge classification system? Why or why not?**

Problems represent one part of the Omaha system. Interventions and targets of nursing care are also classified and organized in this system.

Interventions and Targets

The second level of the Omaha classification scheme is a description of four nursing interventions and 62 target interventions. Nursing interventions are defined as: (1) health teaching, guidance, and counseling; (2) treatments and procedures; (3) case management; and (4) surveillance. The interventions and targets in the Omaha system are broad conceptual categories that help define nursing interventions and label specific foci of nursing care, assessment, planning, intervention, and evaluation. Targets, defined as objects of nursing interventions or nursing activities, are used to delineate a problem-specific intervention category in which an action or activity is directed. Given the ONCS, a nurse selects one or more targets. Targets are then coupled with an intervention category that addresses a specific client problem. Targets are not completely determined, so the category of "other" appears at the end of the list, enabling a nurse to document additional nursing care issues. When selecting interventions, nurses select one of the four major intervention categories. Target actions specify a plan or intervention category directed toward influencing a client's problem. An example of an intervention category of treatments and procedures is "positioning." The definitions of the interventions and a list of targets within the intervention scheme are contained in Boxes 8-2 and 8-3.

BOX 8-2 Intervention Scheme of the Omaha Nursing Classification System

I.   Health Teaching, Guidance, and Counseling

Health teaching, guidance, and counseling are nursing activities that range from giving information, anticipating client problems, and encouraging client action and responsibility for self-care and coping, to assisting with decision making and problem solving. The overlapping concepts occur on a continuum with the variation resulting from the client's self-direction capabilities.

II. Treatments and Procedures

Treatments and procedures are technical nursing activities directed toward preventing signs and symptoms, identifying risk factors and early signs and symptoms, and decreasing or alleviating signs and symptoms.

III. Case Management

Case management includes nursing activities of coordination, advocacy, and referral. These activities involve facilitating service delivery on behalf of the client, communicating with health and human service providers, promoting assertive client communication, and guiding the client toward use of appropriate community resources.

IV. Surveillance

Surveillance includes nursing activities of detection, measurement, critical analysis, and monitoring to indicate client status in relation to a given condition or phenomenon.

Reprinted with permission from Norma M. Lang, PhD, RN, FAAN, FRCN, editor, *Nursing Data Systems: The Emerging Framework* © 1995 American Nurses Publishing, American Nurses Foundation/American Nurses Association, 600 Maryland Avenue, SW, Suite 100W, Washington, DC 20024-2571.

BOX 8-3 Targets for Intervention Activities in the Omaha Nursing Classification

01. Anatomy/physiology
02. Behavior modification
03. Bladder care
04. Bonding
05. Bowel care
06. Bronchial hygiene
07. Cardiac care
08. Caretaking/parenting skills
09. Cast care
10. Communication
11. Coping skills
12. Day care/respite care
13. Discipline
14. Dressing change/wound care
15. Durable medical equipment
16. Education
17. Employment
18. Environment
19. Exercises
20. Family planning
21. Feeding procedures
22. Finances
23. Food
24. Gait training
25. Growth/development
26. Homemaking
27. Housing
28. Interaction
29. Lab findings
30. Legal system
31. Medical/dental care
32. Medication action/side effects
33. Medication administration
34. Medication setup
35. Mobility/transfers
36. Nursing care, supplementary
37. Nutrition
38. Nutritionist
39. Ostomy care
40. Other community resource
41. Personal care
42. Positioning
43. Rehabilitation
44. Relaxation/breathing techniques
45. Rest/sleep
46. Safety
47. Screening
48. Sickness/injury care
49. Signs/symptoms—mental/emotional
50. Signs/symptoms—physical
51. Skin care
52. Social work/counseling
53. Specimen collection
54. Spiritual care
55. Stimulation/nurturance
56. Stress management
57. Substance use
58. Supplies
59. Support group
60. Support system
61. Transportation
62. Wellness
63. Other

Reprinted with permission from Norma M. Lang, PhD, RN, FAAN, FRCN, editor, *Nursing Data Systems: The Emerging Framework* © 1995 American Nurses Publishing, American Nurses Foundation/American Nurses Association, 600 Maryland Avenue, SW, Suite 100W, Washington, DC 20024-2571.

Outcomes and Problem Ratings

The individuals who developed the Omaha classification system realized the importance of outcome specification. Attempts to measure and specify outcomes resulted in the development of a select set of outcomes and a problem resolution rating scale. Outcomes in the Omaha classification system are scaled and rated in terms of achievement in three areas: knowledge, behavior, and status. The problem-rating scale for outcomes, designed for use throughout the time of client service, is intended to measure progress in relation to specific problems and to provide both a guide for practice and a method of documentation. When establishing the initial ratings for client problems, the nurse creates a baseline, capturing the condition and circumstances of the client at a given point in time. This admission baseline is used to compare and contrast the client's condition and circumstances. The comparison or change in ratings over time are used to assess client progress in relation to nursing intervention and thus to judge the effectiveness of the care plan. The problem-rating scale for outcomes is the tool used for quantifying client outcomes. The scale consists of ratings in three categories: knowledge, behavior, and status. Rating choices for each outcome are improved, stabilized, or deteriorated. These ratings assist in determination of the problem's severity and also enable the nurse to measure a client's progress during the period of service. This documentation system also enables the nurse to communicate client progress to others (Martin & Scheet, 1995).

The problem-rating scale (see Table 8-1) consists of three subscales. The first is for knowledge, the second for behavior, and the third for status. Each scale has a rating associated with it (1 = no knowledge and 5 = superior knowledge). The scale does not include a formal set of questions that can be scored and summed to produce a final numeric rating. Instead, nurses are expected to have a knowledge base and the clinical judgment skills that allow them to determine a score or rating for achievements of outcomes or problem resolution in the areas of knowledge, behavior and status of the problem (Martin & Scheet 1992).

An advantage of the Omaha system is that it provides standardization of the framework and structure for documenting care in community contexts. Standard language provides useful information for clinical decision making and facilitates continuity of care among and across agencies. The Omaha system facilitates management of clinical data in the areas of public health, home health, and ambulatory care centers. The major strengths of the system are the relevant labels for problems. There are specific defined interventions coupled with a means for measuring achievement of the status of outcomes.

Some of the limitations of the Omaha system are its problem-oriented focus. Embedded in the system is a medical model body system that limits reasoning about other issues and nursing diagnoses. The outcomes in the context of the system are general rather than specific.

CASE STUDY: MS. BESSIE LEE'S STORY

Ms. Bessie Lee is a 77-year-old African-American woman. She is in relatively good health. She has glaucoma in both eyes and is legally blind. She has insulin-dependent diabetes mellitus (IDDM). A nurse comes in and prepares her insulin shots which Ms. Lee gives to herself. Ms. Lee has a neighbor who takes her vital signs and makes her breakfast every morning. Ms. Lee is unable to make her own meals because she is unable to see well enough. Because she has trouble preparing her food, she eats very little and the visiting nurse is concerned about her calorie intake.

TABLE 8-1   **Problem-Rating Scale for Outcomes in the Omaha Nursing Classification System**

OUTCOME/ CONCEPT	1	2	3	4	5
Knowledge: the ability of the client to remember and interpret information	No knowledge	Minimal knowledge	Basic knowledge	Adequate knowledge	Superior knowledge
Behavior: the observable responses, actions, or activities of the client fitting the occasion or purpose	Not appropriate	Rarely appropriate	Inconsistently appropriate	Usually appropriate	Consistently appropriate
Status: the condition of the client in relation to objective and subjective defining characteristic	Extreme signs/ symptoms	Severe signs/ symptoms	Moderate signs/ symptoms	Minimal signs/ symptoms	No signs/ symptoms

Reprinted with permission from Norma M. Lang, PhD, RN, FAAN, FRCN, editor, *Nursing Data Systems: The Emerging Framework* © 1995 American Nurses Publishing, American Nurses Foundation/American Nurses Association, 600 Maryland Avenue, SW, Suite 100W, Washington, DC 20024-2571.

STOP AND THINK

1. If you were Ms. Lee's nurse, how would you reason about her needs and care?

2. Based on the information in the clinical vignette and a review of the problem classification listed in Box 8-1, what problems do Ms. Lee and the nurse have to tackle?

3. Based on data from the story, what outcomes are important in terms of knowledge, behavior, and status?

4. How might the OPT model assist you in structuring and reasoning about outcomes that would be important in this case?

5. How does the Omaha system help you reason about the problems, interventions, and outcomes important to this case?

SPINNING AND WEAVING THE CLINICAL REASONING WEB

The nurse uses the Omaha classification system as the taxonomy to structure and give meaning to the cues as she reasons, spins, and weaves a Clinical Reasoning Web. Remember, clinical reasoning presupposes that you have done the reading, memorizing, drilling, writing, and practicing necessary to gain the clinical vocabulary of the classification system in order to interpret data from the client story. In this case, such knowledge work includes being familiar with the Omaha system and the targets for nursing intervention. Fundamental knowledge needed to plan care for Ms. Lee includes knowledge about the pathophysiology of diabetes, glaucoma, and the physiological, psychological, and sociological sequelae of aging. Fundamental knowledge in these areas helps support clinical reasoning. Spinning and weaving the web involves the use of several thinking strategies in order to determine the keystone issue that is likely to benefit from intervention and influence many of the health care issues and concerns that have been identified. The thinking strategies of self-talk, schema search, prototype identification, hypothesizing, and if–then thinking support the nurse as relationships in the Clinical Reasoning Web are established. Table 8-2 serves as an example of these relationships.

THINKING STRATEGIES THAT SUPPORT REFLECTIVE CLINICAL REASONING

It is difficult to generate diagnostic hypotheses for Ms. Lee's case if one does not know the definitions, classifications, and categories of diagnoses associated with the

---

TABLE 8-2 Omaha Nursing Classification Domains, Data, and Problems in Ms. Bessie Lee's story

DOMAIN	DATA	PROBLEM
Environmental	77-year-old lives alone	Lives alone, low income
Psychosocial	Isolated at home because of visual impairment	Social contact
Physiological	Legally blind, secondary to diabetes	Vision, safety, physical activity
Health-Related Behavior	Does not eat regularly	Nutrition
	Needs supervision for medication administration	Prescribed medication regimen
		Technical procedures
		Health care supervision

STOP AND THINK

1. **What are some of the functional relationships among the vision problem, meal preparation, medication administration, dietary intake, and Ms. Lee's nutritional status?**
2. **How will representing these issues in a Clinical Reasoning Web make the relationships more explicit?**
3. **What thinking strategies help in the process?**
4. **What keystone issue emerges from the reasoning activities?**

Omaha system. The thinking strategies of self-talk, schema search, prototype identification, hypothesizing, and if–then thinking support the nurse while creating, spinning, and weaving relationships in the Clinical Reasoning Web.

Self-Talk

Self-talk answers the question, "What are the nursing diagnostic possibilities associated with the issue of an elderly person living alone, who has IDDM and is legally blind, and who has no health care supervision?" Given the Omaha classification system, problems in the domains are fairly well categorized. The answer to this question results in the identification of problems relevant to the case. For example, social contact, communication with community resources, vision, health care supervision and nutrition, and prescribed medication regimen as well as the technical procedures associated with self-administration of insulin provide a focus for the care planning around Ms. Lee's story. While spinning and weaving the Clinical Reasoning Web, one has to think out loud to oneself and reason about the possible nursing diagnoses that are relevant to Ms. Lee's story. Nursing diagnoses that are typical for clients with IDDM and impaired vision are also considered.

Prototype Identification

Prototype identification is use of a model case as a reference point for comparative analysis. Ms. Lee's case is one instance of an elderly woman living alone with a chronic condition, in need of adherence to a medication regimen that requires health care supervision. With prototype identification, one considers the textbook descriptions and explanations of the care needs of clients with diabetes. The prototype is a reference point for comparative analysis. Using knowledge from the prototype helps in thinking about relationships among problems, interventions, and outcomes. The Omaha system provides the structure and terminology to categorize problems and organize the nursing care focus for Ms. Lee in regard to knowledge, behavior, and status outcomes the nurse hopes to influence in her case.

Schema Search

Public health nurses often see clients similar to Ms. Lee. Past clinical experiences are helpful in reasoning about this specific case. Schema search is the process of accessing general and/or specific patterns of past experiences that might apply to the current situation. Based on these clinical experiences, nurses collect repertoires of care patterns that help them add to their clinical reasoning knowledge base. The more experiences one has, the more associations one can make and the greater the understanding in complex cases.

Hypothesizing

Given Ms. Lee's story, explain the set of facts identified in the story. Using the Omaha system, the diagnostic hypotheses or problems become the origins and insertion points for making associations as one develops a Clinical Reasoning Web. As one begins spinning and weaving the web, it is easy to see how the data from this case lead one to identify some hypotheses about the client situation. Figure 8-1 shows the diagnostic hypotheses generated for this case.

The lines indicate there are relationships among IDDM, blindness, vision, physical activity, environmental domain, low-income retiree status, living alone, nutrition, health care supervision, health-related behaviors, prescribed medical regimen, technical procedures, communication with community resources, social contact, psychosocial domain problems, safety, and the physiological domain of the Omaha system problem categories.

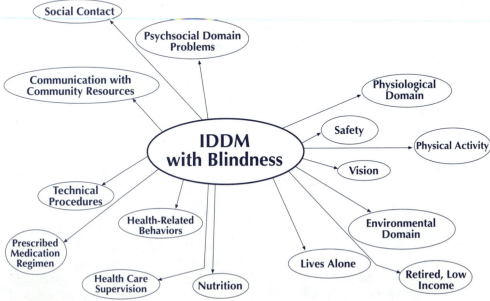

FIGURE 8-1   Beginning the Clinical Reasoning Web for Ms. Bessie Lee

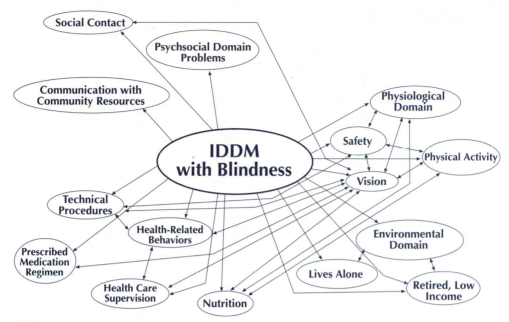

FIGURE 8-2   Developing Relationships in the Ms. Bessie Lee Web

If–Then Thinking

If Ms. Lee has significant visual impairment, then she will have difficulty with health-related behavior of nutrition, safety, technical procedures, social contact, physiological domain problems, physical activity, and environmental domain problems. Because of all of these relationships she needs health care supervision. Figure 8-2 shows the web with these relationships drawn.

Using knowledge from prototype identification of a typical client with circumstances similar to Ms. Lee's the nurse will be alert to safety issues. Safety may be an issue because of living alone, impaired physical activity, physiological parameters, technological procedures, or environmental risks. Look at Figure 8-3 and see how these relationships continue to fill the web.

Figure 8-3 is a completed Clinical Reasoning Web for Ms. Lee. Additional relationships have been identified. With Ms. Lee's low income, she may have difficulty with nutrition, which requires communication with community resources. Since she lives alone, she may have deficits with social contacts, which can cause problems in the psychosocial domain. As the nurse reasons about relationships and draws lines of association and connection on the web, there seems to be a convergence of functional relationships around the keystone issue of nutrition. Doesn't it make sense that if Ms. Lee maintains her nutrition her diabetes will be better controlled, she will have more energy for activity, and safety will not be so compromised? There are a number of ways to frame the data from this case study. Because Ms. Lee has vision problems,

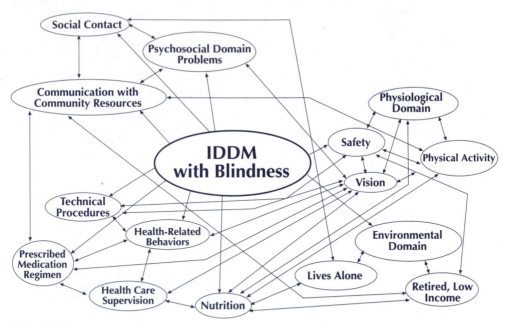

FIGURE 8-3 Clinical Reasoning Web for Ms. Bessie Lee

lives alone, has safety issues, and has diabetes with a complicated medical regimen, it follows that her story can be framed in terms of health care supervision.

Comparative Analysis

Once diagnostic hypotheses and their relationships are made explicit using the web, comparative analysis determines which of these relationships is the keystone or the central supporting issues of Ms. Lee's nursing care focus. Identification of keystone issues enables one to clarify the problem, target, and intervene. For example, managing Ms. Lee's nutrition more effectively contributes to health maintenance in other areas of her life. Identification of these issues help frame the reasoning tasks and determine the test that will fill the evidence gap needed to make clinical judgments.

Health care supervision is one possible frame for Ms. Lee's case. Once a frame has been identified, the stage is set for clarification of the present state and outcome state. The gap between the outcome state and the present state sets up a test. Evidence that will fill the gap will stimulate decision making or choices of nursing interventions that are targeted toward outcome achievement.

Health-seeking behavior is the frame or backdrop of Ms. Lee's story. Given the fact that the Omaha system has three outcomes related to knowledge, behavior, and status, one can begin to generate clinical decision making or specific interventions that will help Ms. Lee make the transition from poor nutrition to adequate intake. Using the thinking strategy of juxtaposing, one can contrast the present state (poor nutrition) with a desired outcome state (1200-calorie American Dietetic Association (ADA) diet.

STOP AND THINK

1. **What theme emerges from creating the Clinical Reasoning Web?**
2. **What present state does the theme suggest?**
3. **Given the present state, what outcome is suggested?**
4. **How does concurrent consideration of outcome state, present state, and frame lead to specification of outcome criteria?**
5. **What is the gap between the present state and outcome state?**
6. **What evidence will fill the gap?**
7. **What clinical decisions does the nurse need to make in order to help Ms. Lee achieve the desired state?**

Juxtaposing

The side-by-side contrast of one state with the other suggests the gap that needs to be filled in order to achieve the outcome. The differences or gaps evident from the present to desired state help establish the creation of a test. Given Ms. Lee's case, the nurse contrasts poor nutritional intake with the desired outcome of a 1200-calorie ADA diet for a person with IDDM. The side-by-side comparison of these two states or conditions creates a gap. The gap from one state to another must be bridged. Bridging the gap is influenced by clinical decisions and nursing actions. In order to meet or match the desired outcome criteria of maintaining a daily 1200-calorie ADA diet, the nurse works with Ms. Lee and the home health aide to make arrangements for insulin injections and design a diet using the resources available to Ms. Lee in the community.

Given the frame of health care supervision and juxtaposing of present state and outcome state, a test between her present state of nutrition and desired outcome state of 1200 calories a day is created. This outcome involves both knowledge and behavior. The outcome according to the Omaha System also includes some measure related

STOP AND THINK

1. **What evidence would you use to know the gap has been filled?**
2. **What nursing care actions or clinical decisions need to be made to obtain the evidence?**
3. **Given the Omaha nursing classification system, what outcomes need to be specified in terms of knowledge, behavior, and status of this problem?**

to status of the problem so changes over time can be noted. These outcomes can then be scaled based on the five point rating scales described in Table 8-1.

Decision Making (Interventions)

To assist Ms. Lee in the transition from the present state of inadequate nutrition to the desired outcome of 1200 calories a day, the nurse activated all four intervention schemes in the Omaha system—health teaching, treatments and procedures, case management, and surveillance. Targets to the intervention scheme included education, nutrition consultation, use of community resources, and support group/system connections. The Omaha classification system provides guidance concerning activities and interventions nurses use to help clients make the transition from identified present states to specified outcomes states. The nurse must decide among an array of possible interventions and targets of interventions. How is the nurse going to assist Ms. Lee in moving from present state to outcome state? The goal of this decision making is to select the interventions and actions that will have the most influence on the outcome and to eliminate interventions and actions that have little or no influence on the outcome. The nurse will know because of comparative analysis and use of the outcome rating scale. Conducting tests involves use of the thinking strategy of comparative analysis and reflexive comparison, and with the Omaha system use of the problem-rating scale as a measure of progress or change. Review the completed OPT Model Worksheet for Ms. Lee in Figure 8-4.

Reflexive Comparison

The next time the nurse comes to see Ms. Lee the nurse will compare her progress from one observation or visit to the next. In this way the nurse is using both the identified outcome criteria and Ms. Lee as her own standard of progress or outcome achievement. The nurse will use reflexive comparison as a way to conduct a test. By juxtaposing the outcome state criteria with a reflexive comparison of Ms. Lee's current state the nurse will have data and evidence that she can use in making a clinical judgment. For example, if Ms. Lee achieved the outcome criteria of maintaining a 1200-calorie diet, she would have achieved the outcome. If however, Ms. Lee's condition deteriorated, reflection and reframing of the keystone issue or the present state would need to take place. This situation would change the story and activate the cue logic and result in a different frame, present state, outcome state, and/or test. A third possibility is that Ms. Lee could improve but not achieve or meet the desired outcome. If this were the case, then reflection about this is likely to provide new data and insights, resulting in another set of clinical decisions or interventions to promote the transition to the outcome state. Data or evidence derived from these comparisons are the facts one uses to make clinical judgments.

On her next visit, Ms. Lee reports that the home health aide who gives her insulin also prepares her breakfast and visits with her while she eats. At noon she gets Meals-on-Wheels service and eats most of her lunch, saving some for dinner. She has also started having a snack before bedtime to get additional calories for the day.

OPT Model Worksheet

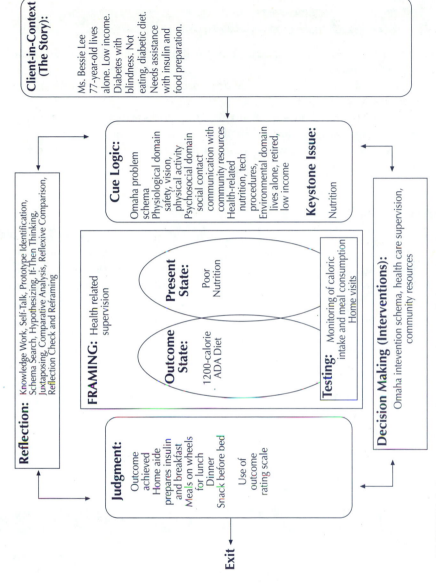

Reflection: Knowledge Work, Self-Talk, Prototype Identification, Schema Search, Hypothesizing, If-Then Thinking, Juxtaposing, Comparative Analysis, Reflexive Comparison, Reflection Check and Reframing

Client-in-Context (The Story):

Ms. Bessie Lee 77-year-old lives alone. Low income. Diabetes with blindness. Not eating, diabetic diet. Needs assistance with insulin and food preparation.

Cue Logic:

Omaha problem schema
Physiological domain
safety, vision, physical activity
Psychosocial domain
social contact
communication with community resources
Health-related
nutrition, tech procedures,
Environmental domain
lives alone, retired, low income

Keystone Issue:

Nutrition

FRAMING: Health related supervision

Outcome State:

1200-calorie ADA Diet

Present State:

Poor Nutrition

Testing: Monitoring of caloric intake and meal consumption Home visits

Judgment:

Outcome achieved
Home aide prepares insulin and breakfast
Meals on wheels for lunch
Dinner
Snack before bed

Use of outcome rating scale

Decision Making (Interventions):

Omaha intevention schema, health care supervision, community resources

Exit

FIGURE 8-4 Completed OPT Model Worksheet for Ms. Bessie Lee

STOP AND THINK

1. Given what Ms. Lee reports, what judgments do you make about outcome achievement?
2. How would this judgment be documented using the Omaha nursing classification system?
3. How did the OPT model and the Omaha system help structure the reasoning and problem identification in this case?
4. Given Ms. Lee's report, do you think it necessary to reframe this situation?

Reframing

What if Ms. Lee did not meet and achieve her desired outcome state criteria? Reframing would be a necessary sequel to this clinical judgment. Reframing is the thinking strategy of attributing a different meaning to the content or context of a situation given a set of cues, tests, decisions, or judgments. If new issues emerged or were not resolved, then reflection would activate cue logic to influence other issues as the nurse continues to reflect and reason about the story. For example, how long will Ms. Lee be able to maintain her independence? What if Ms. Lee developed an ulcer on one of her lower extremities?

Reflection Check

A reflection check pinpoints what has been done correctly; it also identifies errors and provides insights and opportunities to identify and understand how to fix errors or reframe issues.

Use the Thinking Strategies Worksheet in Table 8-3 to record your examples from Ms. Lee's story.

STOP AND THINK

1. If you were Ms. Lee's home health nurse, how would you reason differently about her story? Explain how past clinical experiences would influence your reasoning in this case.
2. Given this case and the Omaha classification system, describe instances of your own use of self-talk, schema search, prototype identification, hypothesizing, if–then thinking, comparative analysis, juxtaposing, reflexive comparison, reframing, and reflection checking.
3. How will experience with this case influence future clinical reasoning if you encounter a client with a similar story?

TABLE 8-3   Thinking Strategies Worksheet

THINKING STRATEGY	DEFINITION	EXAMPLE FROM MS. LEE'S CASE
Knowledge Work	Active use of reading, memorizing, drilling, writing, reviewing research, and practicing to learn clinical vocabulary	
Self-Talk	Expressing one's thoughts to one's self	
Schema Search	Accessing general and/or specific patterns of past experiences that might apply to the current situation	
Prototype Identification	Using a model case as a reference point for comparative analysis	
Hypothesizing	Determining an explanation that accounts for a set of facts that can be tested by further investigation	
If–Then Thinking	Linking ideas and consequences together in a logical sequence	
Comparative Analysis	Considering the strengths and weaknesses of competing alternatives	
Juxtaposing	Putting the present-state condition next to the outcome state in a side-by-side contrast	
Reflexive Comparison	Constantly comparing the client's state from time of observation to time of observation	
Reframing	Attributing a different meaning to the content or context of a situation based on tests, decisions, or judgments	
Reflection Check	Self-examination and self-correction of critical thinking skills and thinking strategies that support clinical reasoning	

SUMMARY

In this chapter nursing care with a client in a community context was discussed. The Omaha Classification system provided the content for reasoning about problems, interventions, and outcomes in community health contexts. The Omaha classification system was derived from a practice base and has been used and developed over a 20-year period. Advantages of the system include categories for problems, interventions, and outcomes. The system handles most problems that occur in community and home health situations. The problem-rating scale, while general, underscores the importance of focusing on outcomes in the areas of knowledge, behavior, and status of identified conditions. Disadvantages of the system relate to its interface with other knowledge development work in nursing. The OPT model helps structure reasoning using Omaha content given a client's story. Thinking strategies that support clinical reasoning in general are also useful in the context of community care.

KEY CONCEPTS

1. Health care is moving into the community. Some people suggest community care is the crux of professional nursing education and practice.
2. The Omaha classification system is a practice-based classification system that consists of problem domains, interventions, and outcomes.
3. Combining the Omaha system and the OPT model provides structure for reasoning about client care needs in community contexts.

STUDY QUESTIONS AND ACTIVITIES

1. Consider your own community health clinical experiences. What classification systems do the home health nurses in your community use? Why were these systems chosen? What are the advantages and disadvantages of these systems given the current state of classification system development?
2. Review Ms. Lee's case. How would you spin and weave a Clinical Reasoning Web for her if you had used another classification system, for example, Gordon's functional health patterns or specific NANDA diagnoses?
3. Compare and contrast the nursing interventions and targets of the Omaha system with the categories and definitions of the NIC classification system.
4. Pretend you are a nurse in a community health center that does not use the Omaha nursing classification system. Create an argument for its adoption in your agency. Be sure to explain the value of a knowledge classification system for professional practice as well as quality client care.

REFERENCES

Bezold, C., & Mayer, E. (1996). *Future care: Responding to the demand for change*. New York: Faulkner & Gray.

Clarke, P., & Cody, W. (1994). Nursing theory-based practice in the home and community: The crux of professional nursing education. *Advances in Nursing Science, 17*(2):41–53.

Donaldson, M., Yordy, K., Lohr, K., & Vanselow, N. (Eds.) (1996). *Community care: America's health in a new era*. Washington, DC: National Academy Press.

Henry, S., & Costantino, M. (1997). Classification systems and integrated information systems: Building blocks for transforming data into nursing knowledge. In J. McCloskey & H. Grace (Eds.), *Current issues in nursing* (5th ed., pp. 75–87). St. Louis, MO: Mosby.

Martin, K., Leak, G., & Alden, C. (1992). A research based model for decision-making. *Journal of Nursing Administration, 22*(11), 47–52.

Martin, K. S., & Scheet, N. J. (1992). *The Omaha system: Applications for community health nursing*. Orlando, FL: Saunders.

Martin, K., & Scheet, N. (1995). The Omaha system: Nursing diagnoses interventions and outcomes. In Norma Lang (Ed.), *Nursing data systems: The emerging framework*. Washington, DC: American Nurses Association Publishing.

Martin, K., Scheet, N., & Stegman, M. (1993). Home health clients: Characteristics, outcomes of care and nursing interventions. *American Journal of Public Health, 83*(12), 1730–1734.

North American Nursing Diagnosis Association. (1996). *Nursing diagnoses: Definitions and classifications, 1997–1998*. Philadelphia, PA: North American Nursing Diagnosis Association.

CHAPTER 9

Clinical Reasoning in Community Mental Health Contexts: Using the OPT Model and *DSM IV*

COMPETENCIES

After completing this chapter, the reader should be able to:

1. Use the OPT model and knowledge from the 4th edition of the *Diagnostic Statistical Manual (DSM-IV)* for structuring the clinical reasoning associated with a specific case study.

2. Explain how the structure of the OPT model and the content of *DSM-IV* support clinical reasoning.

3. Create, spin, and weave a Clinical Reasoning Web from Mr. Harvey Zolar's case study.

4. Develop an OPT Model Worksheet for a client in a mental health context.

5. Explain the thinking strategies that support clinical reasoning given community mental health as the context for reasoning about case studies.

6. Form an opinion on the use of *DSM-IV* and the OPT model to organize thinking and reasoning with clients in a community mental health context.

INTRODUCTION

In this chapter we show how information from the *DSM-IV* can be used with the OPT model. The knowledge contained in the *DSM-IV* is used to reason and plan care for a client with a diagnosis of major depressive disorder. The multi-axial aspects of mental health diagnosis are noted. The *DSM-IV* is helpful in working with clients who have mental disorders. To fully address the nursing care needs of clients in mental health contexts, other nursing knowledge classification systems are useful adjuncts to the use of *DSM-IV*. For example, NANDA and NIC resources help expand reasoning about the nursing care needs required for the client described in this chapter. Nurses should become familiar with *DSM-IV* as the knowledge and information in this classification system is especially useful in working with individuals in a community mental health context.

COMMUNITY MENTAL HEALTH: REASONING WITH CARE

According to the American Nurses Association, psychiatric-mental health nursing is a product of society and a force for social change (ANA, 1994). Most likely there will always be a need for psychotherapy as a way to help people cope. The effects of stress and dysfunctional communication patterns among individuals, groups, families, and organizations take their toll. There is a need to integrate psychosocial care with the needs of the medically ill. Likewise, the mentally ill have medical conditions that need attention and management.

Psychiatric-mental health nurses are often involved with treatment and case management of vulnerable populations such as the homeless and those in rural settings. Box 9-1 outlines the scope of activities that concern mental health nurses who practice in community and mental health contexts (ANA, 1994).

BOX 9-1 Psychiatric-Mental Health Nursing's Phenomenon of Concern

1. The maintenance of optimal health and well-being and the prevention of psychobiologic illness.
2. Self-care limitations or impaired functioning related to mental and emotional distress.
3. Deficits in the functioning of significant biological, emotional, and cognitive systems.
4. Emotional stress or crisis components of illness, pain, and disability.
5. Self-concept changes, developmental issues, and life process changes.

---

continued

6. Problems related to emotions such as anxiety, anger, sadness, loneliness, and grief.

7. Physical symptoms that occur along with altered psychological functioning.

8. Alterations in thinking, perceiving, symbolizing, communication, and decision making.

9. Difficulties in relating to others.

10. Behavioral and mental states that indicate the client is a danger to self or others or has a severe disability.

11. Interpersonal, systemic, sociocultural, spiritual, or environmental circumstances or events that affect the mental and emotional well-being of the individual, family, or community.

12. Symptom management, side effects/toxicities associated with psychopharmacologic intervention and other aspects of the treatment regimen.

Reprinted with permission from American Nurses Association, *A Statement on Psychiatric-Mental Health Clinical Nursing Practice and Standards of Psychiatric-Mental Health Nursing Practice.* © 1994 American Nurses Publishing, American Nurses Foundation/American Nurses Association, 600 Maryland Avenue, SW, Suite 100W, Washington, DC 20024-2571, p. 8.

As one can see, psychiatric-mental health nurses diagnose and treat many conditions in a variety of contexts. Nurses who work in community mental health contexts often place a special emphasis on counseling, self-care activities, psychobiological interventions, health teaching, health promotion, health maintenance, and case management. Standards of care and standards of professional practice guide the clinical decision making of both generalists and specialists in psychiatric-mental health nursing practice. Amid all of these nursing activities, nurses reason about the needs of clients who have mental disorders. One of the major knowledge classification systems nurses use in community mental health contexts is the *DSM-IV* published by the American Psychiatric Association.

KNOWLEDGE FOR COMMUNITY MENTAL HEALTH CARE: *DSM-IV*

The *DSM-IV* allows clinicians and researchers to share a universal language in regard to the diagnosis of mental disorders. The universality of this language permits clinicians and researchers to transmit key information through the use of multi-axial diagnoses, and to understand behavioral manifestations of selected mental disorders (Sapp, 1996). The manual presents an atheoretical approach with regard to psychiatric disorders, etiology, or pathophysiological processes (Sapp, 1996; APA, 1994). Each mental disorder is described by diagnostic criteria. These diagnostic criteria have been refined and field tested over many years (APA, 1994). Key features of a *DSM-IV* category diagnosis include a definition of each disorder, descriptive features, associated laboratory findings, associated physical examination facts, and issues to consider given a client's general medical condition. Additional information for each disorder is provided regarding culture and age features, prevalence, course, and data important for differential diagnosis (APA, 1994; Sapp, 1996; Othmer & Othmer, 1994).

Another feature of the *DSM-IV* is the multi-axial assessment format. Five axes provide useful information on these topics:

1. the clinical mental disorder

2. associated personality disorders or issues regarding mental retardation

3. general medical conditions

4. psychosocial and environmental problems

5. global assessments of functioning that relate psychological, social, and occupational functioning based on a hypothetical continuum of mental health and illness (APA, 1994)

DSM-IV also provides a way to document conditions if there is not diagnostic certainty. For example, each diagnostic class has an option called Not Otherwise Specified (NOS). This category is used when the symptom picture is atypical, the symptoms lead to a pattern not included in *DSM-IV,* there is uncertainty about diagnostic conclusions, or there are not enough data to make a decision (APA, 1994).

In 1995 a Primary Care Version of *DSM-IV* (APA, 1995)—*DSM-IV-PC*—was created. This effort was designed as a way to improve communication among primary care providers and mental health professionals. The manual was to be user-friendly and was to have clinical usefulness, educational relevance, compatibility with other coding systems, and research relevance. All of the diagnostic codes in the *DSM-IV-PC* were derived from the *DSM-IV,* which in turn are all official *ICD* codes. The *DSM-IV-PC* manual is a quick reference that provides decision trees for common mental disorders seen in primary care contexts. Several other goals of the project were to promote educational, clinical, and research collaboration. While decision trees are useful, it is important for clinicians to attend to the client's story and not merely match signs and symptoms to a set of decisions. Consider the case of Mr. Harvey Zolar.

CASE STUDY: MR. HARVEY ZOLAR'S STORY

Mr. Harvey Zolar is a 39-year-old white male who has come to the mental health center seeking treatment. He has a history and diagnosis of major depression. However, he is currently seeking treatment for suicidal ideation. He has had two previous hospitalizations. He is currently unemployed and on disability. He reports a 20-pound weight loss in the past three months, inability to sleep at night, and feelings of fatigue. He states, "I cannot get out of my slump." He has, in the past three days, considered suicide. He threatens to slash his wrists with a razor that his deceased father left him. He has no support network other than the people at the mental health center. He has run out of his antidepressant medication, and he decided to buy alcohol with his disability check rather than refill his prescription. He appears unkempt, his hair is dirty and he smells of alcohol and body odor. He sits in the intake office crying softly and muttering that his life is a failure and he has many regrets. The nurse admits Mr. Zolar to the emergency stabilization unit at the mental health center and begins the process of reasoning about his nursing care needs.

STOP AND THINK

1. **If you were Mr. Zolar's nurse, where would you begin to reason about his needs and care?**
2. **Based on the clinical vignette and a review of types of information on the five axes of the *DSM-IV*, what diagnostic hypotheses come to your mind?**
3. **What do you imagine a Clinical Reasoning Web for Mr. Zolar will look like?**
4. **How will the *DSM-IV* help you reason about the problems, interventions, and outcomes important to this case?**
5. **Will knowledge from the *DSM-IV* be sufficient to help plan nursing care for Mr. Zolar?**
6. **How will the OPT model help structure reasoning about this story?**
7. **What outcomes are important in this case?**

SPINNING AND WEAVING THE CLINICAL REASONING WEB

The intake nurse begins the process of creating a Clinical Reasoning Web for Mr. Zolar. The nurse uses both the *DSM-IV* and NANDA as the taxonomy to structure and give meaning to the cues, and to spin and weave a Clinical Reasoning Web. While *DSM-IV* is useful for diagnosing a mental disorder, the nursing care consequences associated with the mental disorder need to be derived from nursing knowledge classification systems. Clinical reasoning presupposes knowledge work. Fundamental knowledge needed to plan care for Mr. Zolar includes knowledge about the psychophysiology of depression and substance abuse, and the ramifications of these diseases intrapersonally and interpersonally. Spinning and weaving the web involves the use of several thinking strategies in order to determine the keystone issue that is likely to benefit from intervention and influence the nursing care issues identified. Thinking strategies of self-talk, schema search, prototype identification, hypothesizing, and if–then thinking support reasoning.

Based on knowledge of the *DSM-IV*, the nurse looks to the criteria for major depressive episode to guide the reasoning about whether Mr. Zolar meets the specific criteria for this condition. This is an instance of prototype identification because the *DSM-IV* criteria are prototypes of the various mental disorders. In this instance, the nurse is matching to a standard and looking for a match or deviations given the facts of Mr. Zolar's story. Mr. Zolar's story is complex because substance abuse is also an issue. Refer to Boxes 9-2 and 9-3 to review the *DSM-IV* criteria for major depressive episode and substance abuse.

BOX 9-2 *DSM-IV* Criteria for Major Depressive Disorder

A. Five (or more) of the following symptoms have been present during the same two-week period and represent a change from previous functioning: at least one of the symptoms is either (1) depressed mood or (2) loss of interest or pleasure.

Note: Do not include symptoms that are clearly due to a general medical condition, or mood-incongruent delusions or hallucinations.

(1) depressed mood most of the day, nearly every day, as indicated by either subjective report (e.g., feels sad or empty) or observation made by others (e.g., appears tearful). *Note:* In children and adolescents, can be irritable mood.

(2) markedly diminished interest or pleasure in all, or almost all, activities most of the day, nearly every day (as indicated by either subjective account or observation made by others).

(3) significant weight loss when not dieting or weight gain (e.g., a change of more than 5% of body weight in a month), or decrease or increase in appetite nearly every day. *Note:* In children, consider failure to make expected weight gains.

(4) insomnia or hypersomnia nearly every day.

(5) psychomotor agitation or retardation nearly every day (observable by others, not merely subjective feelings of restlessness or being slowed down).

(6) fatigue or loss of energy nearly every day.

(7) feelings of worthlessness or excessive or inappropriate guilt (which may be delusional) nearly every day (not merely self-reproach or guilt about being sick).

(8) diminished ability to think or concentrate, or indecisiveness, nearly every day (either by subjective account or as observed by others).

(9) recurrent thoughts of death (not just fear of dying), recurrent suicidal ideation without a specific plan, or a suicide attempt or a specific plan for committing suicide.

continued

B. The symptoms do not meet criteria for a mixed episode.

C. The symptoms cause clinically significant distress or impairment in social, occupational, or other important areas of functioning.

D. The symptoms are not due to the direct physiological effects of substance (e.g., a drug of abuse, a medication) or a general medical condition (e.g., hypothyroidism).

E. The symptoms are not better accounted for by bereavement, i.e., after the loss of a loved one, the symptoms persist for longer than two months or are characterized by marked functional impairment, morbid preoccupation with worthlessness, suicidal ideation, psychotic symptoms, or psychomotor retardation.

Reprinted with permission from the *Diagnostic and Statistical Manual of Mental Disorders,* Fourth Edition. Copyright 1994 American Psychiatric Association.

BOX 9-3 *DSM-IV* Criteria for Substance Abuse

A. A maladaptive pattern of substance use leading to clinically significant impairment or distress, as manifested by one (or more) of the following occurring within a 12-month period:

(1) recurrent substance use resulting in a failure to fulfill major role obligations at work, school, or home (e.g., repeated absences or poor work performance related to substance use; substance-related absences, suspensions, or expulsions from school; neglect of children or household).

(2) recurrent substance use in situations in which it is physically hazardous (e.g., driving an automobile or operating a machine when impaired by substance use).

(3) recurrent substance-related legal problems (e.g., arrests for substance-related disorderly conduct).

(4) continued substance use despite having persistent or recurrent social or interpersonal problems caused or exacerbated by the effects of the substance (e.g., arguments with spouse about consequences of intoxication, physical fights).

B. If the symptoms have never met the criteria for substance dependence for this class of substance disorders considered in the overall diagnostic evaluation using *DSM-IV*.

Reprinted with permission from the *Diagnostic and Statistical Manual of Mental Disorders,* Fourth Edition. Copyright 1994 American Psychiatric Association.

Based on Mr. Zolar's story the nurse recognizes human response consequences that can be treated within the domain of independent nursing practice. So as an adjunct to *DSM-IV,* the nurse also reasons using diagnoses approved for testing by NANDA (1996). Given Mr. Zolar's story, the nurse organizes human response patterns, supporting data, and diagnostic hypotheses for him.

THINKING STRATEGIES THAT SUPPORT REFLECTIVE CLINICAL REASONING

It is difficult to generate diagnostic hypotheses for Mr. Zolar's case if one does not know the definitions, classifications, and categories of diagnoses associated with *DSM-IV* and NANDA. Other knowledge needed to plan care for Mr. Zolar includes knowledge about physiological, psychological, and sociological issues related to depression and substance abuse. Knowledge about ways of coping with chronic mental illness, access and use of community resources, importance of medication compliance, indicators of suicide, and suicide prevention measures are important in this case. The thinking strategies of self-talk, schema search, prototype identification, hypothesizing, and if–then thinking help in the creation and analysis of a Clinical Reasoning Web and completion of an OPT Model Worksheet.

Self-Talk

Self-talk answers the question, "What are the nursing diagnostic possibilities and consequences associated with major depression?" The answer to this question results in the identification of many diagnostic hypotheses. Through the use of self-talk the nurse reasoned by posing the question, "Given the story, what possible nursing diagnoses are associated with each of the nine human response patterns?" Answers to this question reveal possibilities like social isolation, impaired social interaction, self-care deficit, high risk for injury, risk for violence directed toward self, fatigue, sleep pattern disturbance, ineffective individual coping, chronic low self-esteem, knowledge deficit, altered role performance, fear, and anxiety. These diagnoses become the basis for critically thinking about relationships among issues and concerns. Table 9-1 lists the NANDA patterns and possible diagnoses based on the data from Mr. Zolar's story. Figure 9-1 shows the beginning of Mr. Zolar's Clinical Reasoning Web.

PROTOTYPE IDENTIFICATION

Mr. Zolar's case represents one instance of the prototypical depressed client. Knowing what the typical client with major depression experiences enables one to better compare Mr. Zolar's situation with the prototype. Prototypes serve as one standard of care to use as a reference point for comparative analysis. Nursing care issues for depressed clients with suicidal ideation involve risk management and suicide prevention as well as self-care, medication compliance, and emotional and social support. Because of the complexity of the case, more than one prototype might be needed to effectively reason about the fact pattern presented. For example, the prototypes

TABLE 9-1 Human Response Patterns, Data, and Hypotheses from Mr. Harvey Zolar's story

HUMAN RESPONSE PATTERN	DATA	DIAGNOSTIC HYPOTHESIS
Pattern 1: Exchanging	20-pound weight loss	Altered nutrition less than body require-ments
Pattern 2: Communicating	No data	
Pattern 3: Relating	No support systems Unemployed	Impaired social interaction Social isolation Altered role perfor-mance
Pattern 4: Valuing	Expresses regrets	Potential for enhanced spiritual well-being
Pattern 5: Choosing	Destructive thoughts Not taking medications	Ineffective individual coping Noncompliance (medication)
Pattern 6: Moving	Complaints of fatigue, inability to sleep, unkempt appearance (dirty hair and body odor) Inability to manage health Seeking assistance from mental health center	Fatigue Sleep pattern disturbance Altered health maintenance Self-care deficit (grooming)
Patter 7: Perceiving	"I am in a slump" Mutters life is a failure, so many regrets	Chronic low self-esteem Hopelessness Powerlessness
Pattern 8: Knowing	Inadequate follow-through on medication regimen	Knowledge deficit
Pattern 9: Feeling	Suicidal thoughts, plans to slash wrists	Risk for violence directed at self Risk for self-mutilation Anxiety Fear

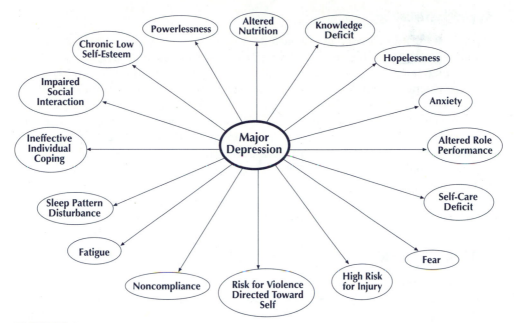

FIGURE 9-1   Beginning the Clinical Reasoning Web for Mr. Harvey Zolar

related to substance use and abuse might be considered relevant. The complexities of dually diagnosed clients in community mental health contexts is a complicated issue in mental health care. Even though Mr. Zolar presented with obvious alcohol and substance use, what issue is of most concern? You gain information about prototypes from reading and studying reference materials, current nursing research literature, and textbooks.

Schema Search

Chances are the nurse in this community mental health center has a repertoire of experiences that include situations similar to Mr. Zolar's story. If experience is present, it supports and enhances the reasoning process. The more experiences one has, the more associations and connections one can make.

STOP AND THINK

1. **Have you had experiences with a client similar to Mr. Zolar?**
2. **What do you know about depressed, suicidal clients who also suffer from a substance use problem?**
3. **What is the priority nursing care issue in your mind as you consider all the possibilities?**

Hypothesizing

When spinning and weaving the Clinical Reasoning Web one has to think out loud and reason about the possible relationships and connections among diagnostic hypotheses. For example, during self-talk, diagnoses are matched with cues or criteria from the *DSM-IV* and NANDA, and preliminary thoughts about diagnostic hypotheses emerge. The diagnostic hypotheses become the origins and insertion points for making associations as one develops a Clinical Reasoning Web. In Mr. Zolar's case, the diagnostic hypotheses are: self-care deficit, knowledge deficit, fatigue, risks for injury and violence to self, sleep patten disturbance, chronic low self-esteem, ineffective individual coping, altered role performance, impaired social interaction, anxiety, fear, hopelessness, powerlessness, and altered nutrition—less than body requirement. Given the large number of nursing diagnoses one could become scattered in care planning. It is more efficient and effective to consider relationships among the possibilities using if–then thinking strategies.

If–Then Thinking

The nurse reasons that there are relationships among chronic low self-esteem, impaired social interaction, anxiety, hopelessness, powerlessness, and risk for violence to self. There are also relationships among ineffective individual coping, noncompliance, and risk for violence directed toward self. Figure 9-2 displays these relationships in the web.

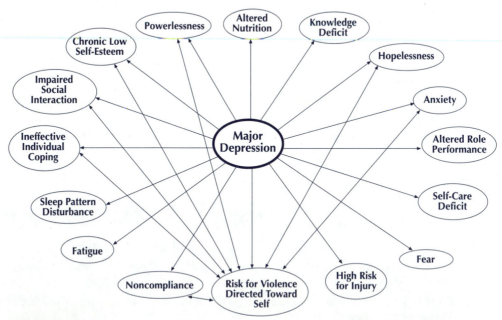

FIGURE 9-2 Developing Relationships in the Mr. Harvey Zolar Web

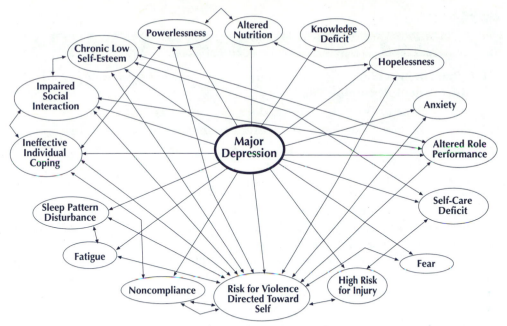

FIGURE 9-3   Clinical Reasoning Web for Mr. Harvey Zolar

Mr. Zolar's case is complex and the completed web in Figure 9-3 demonstrates this complexity.

There are many other relationships between and among the diagnostic hypotheses. Powerlessness, hopelessness, and self-care deficit are related. Noncomplicance is related to ineffective individual coping; sleep pattern disturbance and fatigue are related; and chronic low self-esteem is related to altered role performance. There are a number of other diagnostic hypotheses that have very few connections, For example, knowledge deficit, altered nutrition, fatigue, and fear represent possible diagnostic hypotheses that are not playing a very big part in Mr. Zolar's current situation. However, as the story changes these diagnoses may gain importance. As you look at the web it is clear that there is a convergence toward risk for violence toward self. Thus the issue of safety emerges as a significant focus for immediate attention and is the keystone issue. With this keystone issue and the other data present in the story, one way to frame the thinking task is around the issues of psychological and physical safety.

Comparative Analysis

Identifying the keystone issue enables the nurse to focus care. Once a keystone issue is identified, it has a domino effect. For example, if Mr. Zolar's depression and risk for violence to self is treated, other identified issues, such as self-care deficit, chronic low self-esteem, impaired social interaction, hopelessness, powerlessness, altered role performance, and sleep pattern disturbance are also influenced.

STOP AND THINK

1. **What themes and significant relationships emerge from analysis of the Clinical Reasoning Web?**
2. **What frame and keystone issue does the web suggest?**
3. **Given the keystone issue and present state, what outcomes are suggested?**

Analysis of the Clinical Reasoning Web suggests safety is one theme or frame for Mr. Zolar's case. In many instances of depression, suicide prevention is an overriding concern. Safety is the best choice for the frame because both physiological and psychological safety issues are involved. Specifically, the nurse wants to protect Mr. Zolar from psychological pain and suicide; there is also the issue of safety given the possibility of alcohol withdrawal. Therefore, nursing interventions addressing the keystone issue in this case are organized around the frame of safety with high risk for self-directed violence becoming the keystone issue.

STOP AND THINK

1. **How does the frame influence reasoning about the outcome?**
2. **What influence does the frame have on identification of the present state?**
3. **What criteria will be developed to measure outcome achievement?**
4. **What gap is created between outcome state and the present state?**
5. **How does the side-by side comparison of these two states influence decision making and judgments?**

Since safety is the frame or backdrop of Mr. Zolar's story, an appropriate outcome based on reflection and analysis of the web is risk reduction in regard to self-directed violence as evidenced by improved mood and elimination of suicidal ideation in favor of positive thinking. Using the strategy of juxtaposing, the contrast between the present state of risk for self-directed violence and desired state of improved mood with reduced or no suicidal ideation and the development of positive self-talk creates a gap that must be bridged.

Juxtaposing

The side-by-side contrast of one state with the other illustrates the differences between the two states. The differences or gaps evident from the present to desired state help establish the conditions for the creation of a test. Evidence derived from test conditions and reflexive comparisons help decision making and judgment. Examine the OPT Model Worksheet in Figure 9-4.

OPT Model Worksheet

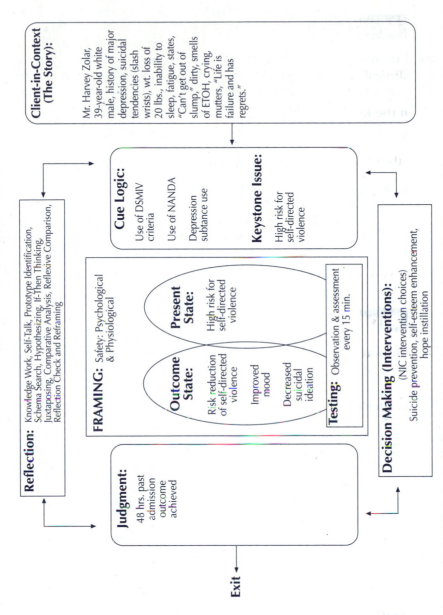

Reflection: Knowledge Work, Self-Talk, Prototype Identification, Schema Search, Hypothesizing, If-Then Thinking, Juxtaposing, Comparative Analysis, Reflexive Comparison, Reflection Check and Reframing

Client-in-Context (The Story):

Mr. Harvey Zolar, 39-year-old white male, history of major depression, suicidal tendencies (slash wrists), wt. loss of 20 lbs., inability to sleep, fatigue, states, "Can't get out of slump," dirty, smells of ETOH, crying, mutters, "Life is failure and has regrets."

Cue Logic:

Use of DSMIV criteria

Use of NANDA

Depression subtance use

Keystone Issue:

High risk for self-directed violence

FRAMING: Safety: Psychological & Physiological

Present State:

High risk for self-directed violence

Outcome State:

Risk reduction of self-directed violence

Improved mood

Decreased suicidal ideation

Testing: Observation & assessment every 15 min.

Decision Making (Interventions):
(NIC intervention choices)
Suicide prevention, self-esteem enhancement, hope instillation

Judgment:

48 hrs. past admission outcome achieved

Exit

FIGURE 9-4 Completed OPT Model Worksheet for Mr. Harvey Zolar

In Mr. Zolar's case, the nurse contrasts high risk for self-directed violence with the desired outcome of improved mood and reduced suicidal ideation. The side-by-side comparison of these two states results in a gap. The gap must be bridged from one state to the other. In order to meet or match the desired outcome criteria of improved mood and elimination of suicidal ideation, the nurse will make clinical decisions and choose nursing actions and interventions to bridge the gap. As decisions are made and actions applied, the nurse will determine changes in Mr. Zolar's condition. Since the frame for this case is psychological and physiological safety, test evidence based on the juxtaposing of present state and outcomes state will involve data related to his mood state and his thought processes about suicide.

Decision Making (Interventions)

To assist Mr. Zolar in making the transition from the present state of high risk for self-directed violence, the nurse activated clinical decision making related to nursing actions and interventions. NIC is a knowledge classification system that provides guidance concerning activities and interventions nurses use to help clients make the transition from identified present states to specified outcome states. The nurse must decide from among an array of possible interventions. For example, in Part IV of NIC (McCloskey & Bulechek, 1996) there are tables that link NIC interventions to NANDA diagnoses. Review the NIC Interventions outlined in Boxes 9-4, 9-5, and 9-6. Pay close attention to the NANDA diagnosis of high risk for self-directed violence and the NIC interventions for treating that condition. What clinical decisions need to be made in Mr. Zolar's case? For example, surveillance and suicide prevention become the priority nursing interventions in this case. Note also that nursing interventions associated with substance use treatment are linked with the diagnosis of self-directed violence.

Box 9-5 defines the NANDA diagnosis of hopelessness and the suggested nursing interventions for that problem. These interventions consist of hope instillation, mood management, complex relationship building, decision-making support, and sleep enhancement. Specific nursing activities for each of these interventions are detailed in the NIC intervention book. As noted earlier, clinical decision making is the selection of interventions from a repertoire of actions that facilitate the achievement of a desired outcome state.

Box 9-6 identifies nursing interventions that could be used to assist Mr. Zolar with the management of his chronic low self-esteem. For example, use of the interventions of self-esteem enhancement, social support enhancement, and emotional support might be specific clinical decisions the nurse would make.

Reflexive Comparison

The process and goal of clinical decision making is to select the interventions and actions that will have the most influence on the outcome and eliminate interventions and actions that have little or no influence on the outcome. Following the implemen-

BOX 9-4 Nursing Intervention Classification, Definition, and Activities for the Intervention for Violence, High Risk for: Self-Directed or Directed at Others

DEFINITION: A state in which an individual experiences behaviors that can be physically harmful either to the self or others.

SUGGESTED NURSING INTERVENTIONS FOR PROBLEM RESOLUTION:

Abuse Protection
Abuse Protection: Child
Abuse Protection: Elder
Anger Control Assistance
Anxiety Reduction
Area Restriction
Art Therapy
Behavior Management
Behavior Management: Self-Harm
Behavior Modification
Calming Technique:
Coping Enhancement
Crisis Intervention
Delusion Management
Dementia Management
Distraction
Environmental Management: Violence Prevention

Fire-Setting Precautions
Medication Administration
Mood Management
Physical Restraint
Seclusion
Security Enhancement
Substance Use Prevention
Substance Use Treatment
Substance Use Treatment: Alcohol Withdrawal
Substance Use Treatment: Drug Withdrawal
Suicide Prevention
Support System Enhancement
Surveillance
Surveillance: Safety

ADDITIONAL OPTIONAL INTERVENTIONS:

Animal-Assisted Therapy
Behavior Modification: Social Skills
Family Involvement
Family Support
Guilt Work Facilitation
Impulse Control Training
Medication Management

Mutual Goal Setting
Play Therapy
Presence
Reality Orientation
Self-Esteem Enhancement
Support Group

Reprinted with permission from McCloskey, J. C., & Bulechek, G. M. (1996). *Nursing intervention classification* (2nd ed.). St. Louis, MO: Mosby.

tation of decision, the nurse will evaluate progress or state transition using primarily the thinking strategy of reflexive comparison. Reflexive comparison is a thinking strategy that involves constant comparison of the client's state from time of observation to time of observation. For example, compare Mr. Zolar's risk for self-directed violence from one suicide precaution check to the next. In this way, the nurse uses both the

BOX 9-5   Nursing Intervention Classification, Definition, and Activities for the Intervention for Hopelessness

DEFINITION: A subjective state in which an individual sees limited or no alternatives or personal choices available and is unable to mobilize energy on own behalf.

SUGGESTED NURSING INTERVENTIONS FOR PROBLEM RESOLUTION:

Complex Relationship Building
Decision-Making Support
Emotional Support
Energy Management
Hope Instillation
Mood Management

Presence
Reminiscence Therapy
Sleep Enhancement
Socialization Enhancement
Support Group

ADDITIONAL OPTIONAL INTERVENTIONS:

Anger Control Assistance
Animal-Assisted Therapy
Activity Therapy
Cognitive Stimulation
Counseling
Crisis Intervention
Distraction
Exercise Promotion
Exercise Therapy: Ambulation

Grief Work Facilitation
Grief Work Facilitation: Perinatal Death
Music Therapy
Mutual Goal Setting
Client Contracting
Play Therapy
Self-Care Assistance
Spiritual Support
Suicide Prevention

Reprinted with permission from McCloskey, J. C., & Bulechek, G. M. (1996). *Nursing intervention classification* (2nd ed.). St. Louis, MO: Mosby.

STOP AND THINK

1. **What clinical decisions would you make given Mr. Zolar's case?**
2. **How would your clinical decisions promote achievement of the outcomes?**
3. **What evidence would you use to judge outcome achievement?**

identified outcome criteria and Mr. Zolar as his own standard in terms of making judgments about outcome achievement. There are three possible consequences of such testing through reflexive comparison. First, Mr. Zolar could achieve the desired outcome of decreased risk for self-directed violence, increased mood, and a decrease in suicidal ideation. Second, Mr. Zolar's condition could deteriorate, necessitating reflection and reframing of issues, concerns, and facts. This situation would change

---

BOX 9-6   Nursing Intervention Classification, Definition, and Activities for the Intervention for Self-Esteem, Chronic Low

DEFINITION: Long-standing negative self-evaluation/feelings about self or self capabilities.

SUGGESTED NURSING INTERVENTIONS FOR PROBLEM RESOLUTION:

Body Image Enhancement   Self-Esteem Enhancement
Counseling   Socialization Enhancement
Emotional Support   Support System Enhancement

ADDITIONAL OPTIONAL INTERVENTIONS:

Active Listening   Presence
Anxiety Reduction   Role Enhancement
Complex Relationship Building   Suicide Prevention
Coping Enhancement   Support Group
Crisis Intervention   Surveillance: Safety
Decision-Making Support   Therapeutic Touch
Grief Work Facilitation   Values Clarification
Mutual Goal Setting
Pain Management

Reprinted with permission from McCloskey, J. C., & Bulechek, G. M. (1996). *Nursing intervention classification* (2nd ed.). St. Louis, MO: Mosby.

---

the story and activate the cue logic and result in reflection and reframing. Perhaps Mr. Zolar begins to exhibit signs and symptoms of alcohol withdrawal, or he becomes psychotic. Third, Mr. Zolar could improve but not meet the desired outcome.

As an example, 48 hours later, Mr. Zolar's mood is improved and he does not have thoughts of suicide. Since he has reconnected with the community mental health center and his therapist, they have made arrangements for him to attend a medication clinic within the Mental Health Center in order to get his antidepressant regularly. He has also been referred to a local substance abuse program for evaluation and follow-up.

STOP AND THINK

1. **What evidence do you use to know the gap has been filled?**

2. **What nursing care actions or clinical decisions were done to obtain the evidence?**

3. **Given the *DSM-IV,* NANDA, and NIC, which system was most helpful in supporting the reasoning about this case?**

Reframing

Suppose clinical judgments associated with the results of testing were negative and Mr. Zolar did not achieve enhanced mood with a decrease in suicidal ideation. Reframing would be a necessary sequel to this clinical judgment. Reframing is the thinking strategy of attributing a different meaning to the content or context of a situation given a set of cues, tests, decisions, or judgments.

Reflection Check

A reflection check pinpoints what has been done correctly; it also identifies errors and provides insights and opportunities to identify and understand how to fix errors or reframe issues. Review Mr. Zolar's case and complete the Thinking Strategies Worksheet in Table 9-2 to identify examples of thinking strategies you would use if you were reasoning about this story.

STOP AND THINK

1. **If you were Mr Zolar's nurse, how would you reason differently about his story? Explain how past clinical experiences would influence your reasoning about this case.**
2. **Given this case and the *DSM-IV*, describe instances of your own use of self-talk, schema search, prototype identification, hypothesizing, if–then thinking, comparative analysis, juxtaposing, reflexive comparison, reframing, and reflection checking.**
3. **How will experience with this case influence future clinical reasoning when you encounter a client with a similar story?**

SUMMARY

In this chapter we reviewed the knowledge and skills nurses need to practice and care for clients in community mental health care contexts. We discussed the use of *DSM-IV* and NANDA classification systems that support clinical reasoning. We reasoned about the story of Mr. Zolar, a 39-year-old man who has a history of depression mixed with substance use and possible abuse. Using the clinical vocabulary of *DSM-IV*, NANDA, and NIC, we used the Clinical Reasoning Web and OPT Model Worksheet to reason about his care. Thinking strategies that support clinical reasoning were highlighted. We concluded this chapter with an invitation to identify thinking strategies you would use to reason about Mr. Zolar's case.

TABLE 9-2 Thinking Strategies Worksheet for Mr. Harvey Zolar's Story

THINKING STRATEGY	DEFINITION	EXAMPLE FROM HARVEY ZOLAR CASE
Knowledge Work	Active use of reading, memorizing, drilling, writing, reviewing research, and practicing to learn clinical vocabulary	
Self-Talk	Expressing one's thoughts to one's self	
Schema Search	Accessing general and/or specific patterns of past experiences that might apply to the current situation	
Prototype Identification	Using a model case as a reference point for comparative analysis	
Hypothesizing	Determining an explanation that accounts for a set of facts that can be tested by further investigation	
If–Then Thinking	Linking ideas and consequences together in a logical sequence	
Comparative Analysis	Considering the strengths and weaknesses of competing alternatives	
Juxtaposing	Putting the present-state condition next to the outcome state in a side-by-side contrast	
Reflexive Comparison	Constantly comparing the client's state from time of observation to time of observation	
Reframing	Attributing a different meaning to the content or context of a situation based on tests, decisions, or judgments	
Reflection Check	Self-examination and self-correction of critical thinking skills and thinking strategies that support clinical reasoning	

KEY CONCEPTS

1. There will always be a need for psychotherapy for those individuals who suffer from mental disorders. Standards of care and standards of professional practice guide the clinical decision making of both generalists and specialists in psychiatric-mental health nursing practice. Nurses who work in the community mental health context often place a special emphasis on counseling, self-care activities, and psychobiological interventions.

2. The *DSM-IV* is multi-axial assessment. Five axes provide clinically useful information on these factors: (1) the clinical mental disorder; (2) associated personality disorders, or issues regarding mental retardation; (3) general medical conditions; (4) psychosocial and environmental problems; and (5) a global assessment of functioning that considers psychological, social, and occupational functioning based on a hypothetical continuum of mental health and illness.

3. *DSM-IV* allows both clinicians and researchers to share a universal language in the diagnostic area, to transmit key information through the use of multi-axial diagnoses, and to understand behavioral manifestations of selected mental disorders.

4. While use of the *DSM-IV* helps determine specific mental disorders, other nursing knowledge classifications are needed to determine the nursing diagnoses and interventions related to the nursing care needs of clients with specific mental disorders.

5. Using the tools of the Clinical Reasoning Web, OPT Model Worksheet, and Thinking Strategies Worksheet, one can effectively reason about client care needs in the context of community mental health.

STUDY QUESTIONS AND ACTIVITIES

1. Obtain a copy of the most current edition of *DSM-IV* and *DSM-IV-PC*. Compare and contrast the information contained in these two resources. As you review information in a copy of the *DSM-IV-PC,* consider the advantages and disadvantages of using algorithms as diagnostic tools.

2. Revisit the case of Mr. Zolar described in the chapter. What if the nurse determined substance dependence was the frame and present state? How would reasoning about this case be different?

3. Given the fact that the *DSM-IV* is used by other mental health professions, what do you think the advantages and disadvantages of this are for the development of nursing knowledge?

4. What are the patient care consequences if the nurse only uses the *DSM-IV* knowledge system as the clinical vocabulary to reason about client care issues in community mental health contexts?

5. What are some of the ethical and legal responsibilities nurses have in regard

to learning about the use of knowledge classification systems for professional nursing practice?

REFERENCES

American Nursing Association. (1994). *Statement on psychiatric-mental health clinical nursing practice and standards of psychiatric-mental health clinical nursing practice*. Washington, DC: American Nurses Publishing.

American Psychiatric Association. (1994). *Diagnostic and statistical manual of mental disorders* (4th ed.). Washington, DC: American Psychiatric Association Press.

American Psychiatric Association. (1995). *Diagnostic and statistical manual of mental disorders primary care version*. Washington, DC: American Psychiatric Association Press.

McCloskey, J., & Bulechek, G. (1996). *Nursing intervention classification*. St. Louis, MO: Mosby.

North American Nursing Diagnosis Association. (1996). *Nursing diagnoses: Definitions and classifications, 1997–1998*. Philadelphia, PA: North American Nursing Diagnosis Association.

Othmer, E., & Othmer, S. (1994). *The clinical interview using DSM-IV*. Volume 1: *Fundamentals*. Washington, DC: American Psychiatric Association Press.

Sapp, J. (1996). Diagnosis and the *DSM-IV*. In. S. Lego (Ed.), *Psychiatric nursing: A comprehensive reference* (pp. 15–30). Philadelphia, PA: Lippincott.

CHAPTER 10

Clinical Reasoning in a Long-Term Care Context

COMPETENCIES

After completing this chapter, the reader should be able to:

1. Discuss knowledge and skills needed for the practice of gerontological nursing.
2. Use the OPT model, Gordon's functional health patterns, and NANDA to structure and reason about the nursing care needs of a frail elderly person.
3. Create, spin, and weave a Clinical Reasoning Web using information from the Ms. Sara Monroe case study.
4. Explain how the structure of the OPT model supports clinical reasoning.
5. Analyze the thinking strategies that support clinical reasoning and reflect on ways the model can be used with other clients in long-term care settings.

INTRODUCTION

In this chapter the OPT model is applied to a specific client who resides in a long-term care setting. The knowledge and skills one needs to care for elderly clients are presented. Use of the OPT model and NANDA nursing diagnoses is illustrated with information from the story of Ms. Sara Monroe, a frail elderly person who has dementia and arthritis and many nursing care needs. As in previous chapters, the thinking strategies that support reasoning and use of the OPT model are discussed. Reflection on how one can use the OPT model with other clients in long-term care settings is encouraged.

THE CONTEXT OF LONG-TERM CARE

A long-term care facility is both a home to residents and a health care service center. As the American population ages, greater numbers of people will need care in long-term residential facilities. Estimates are that one in five elderly over age 65 will spend time in a nursing facility; for those over 85, the number is one in three (Mezey, Lynaugh, & Cartier, 1989). The context of care influences diagnoses, interventions, and outcomes. For example, Puzicka (1997) identified the following nursing diagnoses as setting-sensitive but especially noteworthy when one considers care of the elderly:

1. diversional activity deficit
2. alterations in health maintenance
3. high risk for injury
4. noncompliance.

Other diagnostic issues that surface in long-term care facilities include diagnosis and treatment of:

1. alterations in bowel and bladder pattern (urinary incontinence)
2. activity intolerance
3. pain
4. impaired skin integrity
5. alterations in nutrition
6. dehydration
7. self-care deficits (Lekan-Rutledge 1997).

Each of these diagnoses presents significant nursing care challenges.

FOCUS ON GERONTOLOGICAL NURSING

Aging is accompanied by many physiological, psychological, and social challenges. Some people age with grace and maintain their vigor and vitality. Other people experience declines in health as they age. The effects of chronic disease often catch up with people. What are your images and experiences with the effects of aging on health? Perhaps you have a parent, grandparent, friend, or relative who lives in a long-term care facility. What thoughts and images come to mind as you think about the special nursing care required for this person? Where and how do you plan to spend your older years? What will be important to you in terms of your health care concerns and nursing care needs? How prepared are you in the area of gerontological nursing?

The goal of gerontological nursing is to help elderly clients function as fully as possible, realizing their highest potential (Bahr, 1994). Additional goals include the promotion of health, compensation for deficits and impairments, and provision of comfort and sustenance. The diagnosis, treatment, and palliation of responses to actual or potential health problems are also foci of gerontological nursing (Matteson, McConnell, & Linton, 1997).

The knowledge and competencies needed to work with the elderly in the long-term care context are challenging. Essential knowledge and competencies for the practice of gerontological nursing are outlined in Boxes 10-1 and 10-2. Nurses who work in long-term care need to have the knowledge and skills outlined in the illustration.

BOX 10-1   Necessary Knowledge for Nursing Practice in Long-Term Care

Nurses need to know about:

The physical, psychological, and social aspects of aging throughout the life span, and the resultant impact on the individual and the family.

The pathophysiology, epidemiology, and treatment of chronic diseases commonly encountered by elderly people and the impact of these disease processes and associated therapeutic regimens on these individuals and their families.

The spectrum of health services available to the elderly in the community and how that relates to the national spectrum of health services.

The signs and symptoms of a typical presentation of disease in the elderly.

The altered pharmacology of drugs in the elderly.

The influence of environmental factors on human performance and health status in the aged.

The impact of ethnicity on responses to aging-related changes, disease, and developmental events.

Specific standards of nursing care for elderly individuals.

Approaches to health promotion and disease prevention in late life.

The range of ethical reasoning frameworks that apply to care of the elderly.

Reprinted with permission from Matteson, M., McConnell, E., & Linton, A. (1997). *Gerontological nursing concepts and practices* (2nd ed.). Philadelphia, PA: W. B. Saunders

BOX 10-2   Necessary Skills for Practice in Long-Term Care

Nurses who work in long-term care need to be skilled in order to:

Utilize research findings from gerontology as well as nursing and the bio-medical and behavioral sciences to inform nursing practice.

Interact effectively with individuals who have sensory loss.

Perform multidimensional assessment of the elderly person using existing standardized tools and individualized approaches.

Function as members of a coordinated multidisciplinary or interdisciplinary team in providing care to the aged.

Implement rehabilitative nursing techniques.

Help clients integrate past life with present.

Include the elderly person and family members in developing goals for nursing care, even if the individual has significant communication or cognitive impairments.

Modify the environment to maximize the elderly person's ability to function independently.

Provide excellent palliative, supportive, and spiritual care for those who are dying.

Counsel the grieving.

Consider ethical dilemmas encountered by elderly people, their kin, and their health care providers.

Help families and communities overcome hostilities toward the elderly.

Participate in professional activities designed to improve health care for the elderly.

Supervise the efforts of paraprofessional and lay caregivers in providing nursing care to the aged.

Teach paraprofessionals, lay caregivers, and the elderly about the impact of the aging process and disease processes on self-care abilities and requisites of elderly persons.

Teach paraprofessionals, lay caregivers, and the elderly techniques to achieve self-care objectives.

Establish developmentally appropriate criteria for evaluation of nursing care.

Reprinted with permission from Matteson, M., McConnell, E., & Linton, A. (1997). *Gerontological nursing concepts and practices* (2nd ed.). Philadelphia, PA: W. B. Saunders

STOP AND THINK

1. As you review the knowledge required and the skills necessary for working in long-term care, how do they differ from those in other contexts?
2. What is especially important when working with the elderly in a long-term care context?
3. What are some of the ethical and legal implications of working with the elderly in a long-term care context?

CASE STUDY: MS. SARA MONROE'S STORY

Ms. Sara Monroe is a resident in a long-term care facility. She has lived at the facility for four years. She is 84 years old, and has dementia and severe arthritis. One daughter and the daughter's three grandchildren are the only family Ms. Monroe has. The family tries to visit once a week. The family is most distressed that Ms. Monroe does not seem to recognize or interact with them when they visit her. The daughter describes her mother as a "shell of a person." She is totally dependent on someone else because she is immobile. She is oriented to person and sometimes to place, yet is confused and has significant memory loss. She believes she is 50 years old. She constantly complains of pain during her daily morning care activities, and she is extremely anxious when being transferred from bed to chair or vice versa. She cries out, "Please don't let me fall," and she also grabs hold of everything and has a hard time letting go. She becomes very agitated when being lifted or moved in the bed. It seems Ms. Monroe was dropped once during a transfer from her bed to the wheelchair and suffered a broken hip. While the hip has healed, she still becomes anxious and fearful during morning care activities and during any transfer episode.

STOP AND THINK

1. If you were Ms. Monroe's nurse, how would you reason about her needs and care?
2. Based on the information in the clinical vignette and a review of the knowledge and skills listed in Boxes 10-1 and 10-2, what is relevant as you begin to reason about Ms. Monroe's situation?
3. Based on data from the story, what outcomes are important?
4. How might the OPT model assist you in structuring and reasoning about outcomes that would be important in this case?
5. What other nursing knowledge classification systems are going to be useful for understanding and planning Ms. Monroe's nursing care?

SPINNING AND WEAVING THE CLINICAL REASONING WEB

The nurse who is reasoning about Ms. Monroe's care has decided to use Gordon's functional health patterns as a way to organize data associated with the story. In Table 10-1 each of Gordon's functional health patterns is paired with data from the story. Diagnostic hypotheses are derived, which become the origin and insertion points in a Clinical Reasoning Web. Thinking strategies are then applied to understand the functional relationships among the concerns. A keystone issue is likely to emerge from this analysis and synthesis.

The cues related to this client's story include a medical diagnosis of arthritis, being immobile, being agitated, impaired memory, complaints of pain, cries of "please don't let me fall and help me," being underweight, poor range of joint motion in lower extremities, disorientation, no physical therapy, being bedridden, clutching, and client states 50 years old when really 84. The most notable cues associated with care for this client included the anxiety, clutching, complaints of pain, agitation, and cries for help not to hurt her when engaged in helping her with activities of daily living.

The nurse created the beginning Clinical Reasoning Web in Figure 10-1.

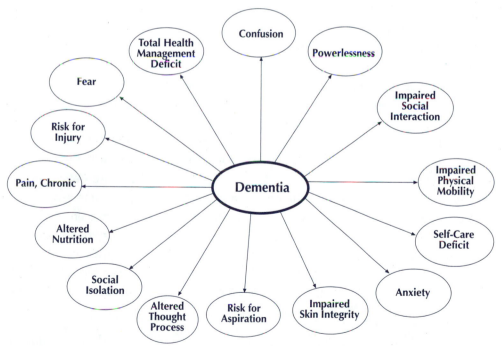

FIGURE 10-1   Beginning Clinical Reasoning Web for Ms. Sara Monroe

TABLE 10-1 Gordon's Functional Health Patterns, Data, and Hypotheses for Ms. Sara Monroe

PATTERN	DATA	DIAGNOSTIC HYPOTHESES
Health perception/health management pattern—client's perceived pattern of health and well-being and how health is managed	Unable to manager her health care needs	Total health management deficit
Nutritional/metabolic pattern—pattern of food and fluid consumption relative to metabolic need and pattern indicators of local nutrient supply	Must be fed, limited range of motion, unable to feed self or maintain fluid intake / Underweight for age and body type	Altered nutrition less than body requirements / At risk for impaired skin integrity
Elimination pattern—patterns of excretory function (bowel, bladder, and skin)	Needs assistance in managing bowel and bladder elimination	
Activity/exercise pattern—pattern of exercise, activity, leisure, and recreation	Limited range of motion / Immobile / No physical therapy / Clutches to nurse upon transfer, will not let go	Fatigue / Impaired physical activity / At risk for injury related to immobility / Self-care deficit, total
Cognitive/perceptual pattern—sensory-perceptual and cognitive pattern	Confused, memory loss / Frequent complaints of pain, especially during transfer to and from wheelchair / States she is 50 even though 84 years old	Anxiety and fear / Chronic pain / Sensory-perceptual alterations / Altered thought process / Confusion

continued

TABLE 10-1 *(continued)*

PATTERN	DATA	DIAGNOSTIC HYPOTHESES
Sleep/rest pattern— patterns of sleep, rest, and relaxation	Rests most of day due to impaired mobility	Alterations in sleep pattern
Self-perception/self-concept pattern— self-concepet pattern and perceptions of self (e.g., body comfort, body image, feeling state)	Appears anxious and frightened Expresses fear when transferring Agitated	Powerlessness Fear Anxiety
Role/relationship pattern— pattern of role-engage-ments and relationships	Daughter and family visit Daughter notes mother is "shell of a person" Mother is unresponsive during visits	Impaired social interaction Impaired verbal communication Social isolateion
Sexuality/reproductive pattern—client's patterns of satisfaction and dissatisfaction with sexuality pattern; describes reproductive patterns	No data	
Coping/stress tolerance pattern—general coping pattern and effective-ness of the pattern in terms of stress tolerance	No data	
Value/belief pattern— patterns of values, beliefs (including spiritual), or goals that guide choices of decisions	No data	

1. What are some of the functional relationships among Ms. Monroe's anxiety and self-care deficit? Fear and risk for injury? Confusion and fear?
2. How will representing these issues in a Clinical Reasoning Web make the relationships more explicit?
3. What thinking strategies help in the process?
4. What keystone issue emerges from the reasoning activities?

THINKING STRATEGIES THAT SUPPORT REFLECTIVE CLINICAL REASONING

It is difficult to generate diagnostic hypotheses for Ms. Monroe's case if one does not know the definitions, classifications, and categories of diagnoses associated with Gordon's functional health patterns and NANDA. Other prerequisite knowledge needed to plan care for Ms. Monroe includes facts about the physiological, psychological, and sociological effects of dementia and arthritis. Understanding about the dynamics of coping with chronic illness in a long-term care facility, normal and abnormal cognitive functioning, growth and developmental needs of the elderly, the psychology of aging, and the special requirement of gerontological nursing clients is also a necessary prerequisite. The Clinical Reasoning Web helps make many of the relationships among these issues evident. Through application of thinking strategies one can reason more effectively about Ms. Monroe's nursing care needs.

Self-Talk

Self-talk answers the question, "What are the nursing care consequences and diagnostic possibilities associated with dementia?" Dementia has many human response consequences. Some of the diagnostic possibilities include: fear, confusion, self-care deficit, anxiety, impaired mobility, social isolation, pain, risk for injury, risk for impaired skin integrity, and altered nutrition—less than body requirement. Ms. Monroe is exhibiting signs and symptoms that could indicate any or all of these problems. Review and analyze the Clinical Reasoning Web for her in Figure 10-2.

Use your knowledge about care of the elderly and think about other diagnostic hypotheses that might be added to the web.

Prototype Identification

What prototype clients help one understand or reason about Ms. Monroe's specific situation? Many prototypes can be used. For example, what are the prototypical nurs-

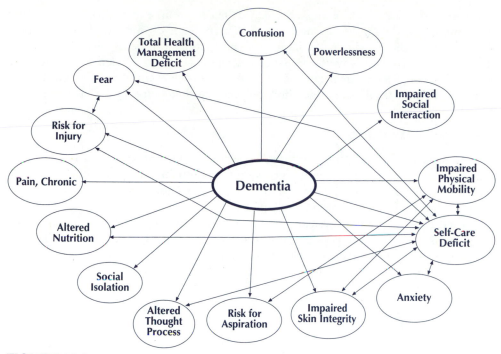

FIGURE 10-2   Developing Relationships in the Ms. Sara Monroe Web

ing care issues for an elderly person, a person with dementia, and someone who has a history of a broken hip? Consulting references that describe the client care needs of people with these conditions helps one reason more effectively about Ms. Monroe's care.

Schema Search

Remembering past clinical experiences with frail elderly clients is a thinking strategy that supports clinical reasoning. For example, experiences may remind you of the fact that most clients with dementia suffer from self-care deficits and often exhibit signs and symptoms of agitation, anxiety, and fear. These emotional states have consequences for interpersonal interactions, social isolation, and risks for injury.

Hypothesizing

Given Ms. Monroe's story, how might one explain the set of cues identified in the story? Using Gordon's functional health patterns as a guide, the following diagnostic hypotheses were generated: total health management deficit, altered nutrition—less than body requirements, at risk for impaired skin integrity, impaired physical activity, at risk for injury related to immobility, total self-care deficit, anxiety, fear, chronic pain, altered thought process, confusion, powerlessness, impaired social interaction, and social isolation. Each of these NANDA diagnoses is an explanation that accounts for some of the data in Ms. Monroe's story. The number of nursing diagnoses possible for elderly clients who live in long-term care settings can be overwhelming. Thus, it is important to identify keystone issues that effectively and efficiently resolve nursing care needs. As one analyzes the web, what keystone issues are evident for Ms. Monroe? If–then thinking is one thinking strategy that helps make clear keystone issues.

If–Then Thinking

As you look at the beginning web for Ms. Monroe, you see a number of diagnoses that relate to physical well-being. For example, confusion, altered thought process, impaired physical mobility, altered nutrition, risk for injury, impaired skin integrity, anxiety, and fear are all related to self-care deficit. There are other relationships that influence care. Impaired physical mobility is related to impaired skin integrity; risk for aspiration is related to impaired physical mobility. And risk for injury is related to fear. Figure 10-2 shows the web with these connections. There are other relationships that complete the web as seen in Figure 10-3.

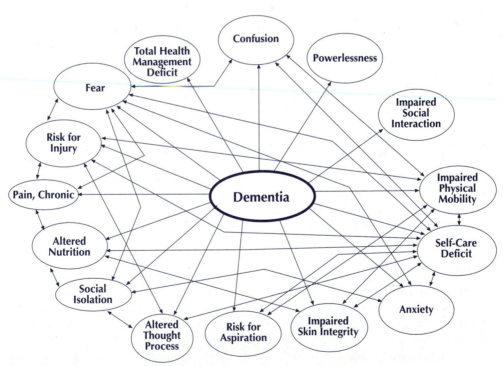

FIGURE 10-3   Clinical Reasoning Web for Ms. Sara Monroe

Comparative Analysis

Once diagnostic hypotheses and their relationships are made explicit using the web, comparative analysis helps determine the keystone or the central supporting issues of Ms. Monroe's nursing care focus. For example, one of the keystone issues in this case is self-care deficit. Self-care deficit is embedded in the larger framework of needs specific to the care of frail elderly clients. This frame organizes many of the nursing care needs associated with this client's story. Self-care deficit requires nursing care resources. Individuals rely on nursing care for feeding, toileting, turning, positioning, social stimulation, skin care, and all activities related to treatment of disuse syndrome. Self-care deficit is also likely to have psychological consequences and influence feelings of hopelessness, powerlessness, anxiety, and fear. Identification of these issues help frame the reasoning tasks and determine the gap between the present state and outcome state.

STOP AND THINK

1. **What theme emerges from analyzing the Clinical Reasoning Web?**
2. **What present state does the theme suggest?**
3. **Given the present state, what outcome is suggested?**
4. **How does concurrent consideration of outcome state, present state, and frame lead to specification of outcome criteria?**
5. **What is the gap between the present state and the outcome state?**
6. **What evidence will fill the gap?**
7. **What clinical decisions does the nurse need to make in order to help Ms. Monroe achieve the desired outcome state?**

Self-care needs of the frail elderly is one possible theme or frame for Ms. Monroe's case. Once a frame has been identified, the stage is set for clarification of the present state and outcome state. The gap between the outcome state and the present state sets up a test. Evidence that will fill the gap will stimulate decision making or choices of nursing interventions that are targeted toward outcome achievement. See Figure 10-4 for the OPT Model Worksheet for Ms. Monroe.

Since self-care needs of the frail elderly is the frame or backdrop of Ms. Monroe's story, a self-care deficit with agitation is the present state, and the desired outcome is self-care maintenance with decrease in agitation and anxiety or an increase in comfort. Using the thinking strategy of juxtaposing, one can contrast the two states and begin to see the gaps that exist. One can then begin to make clinical decisions about specific interventions that will help Ms. Monroe make the transition from states of anxiety and agitation to greater comfort and self-care maintenance.

OPT Model Worksheet

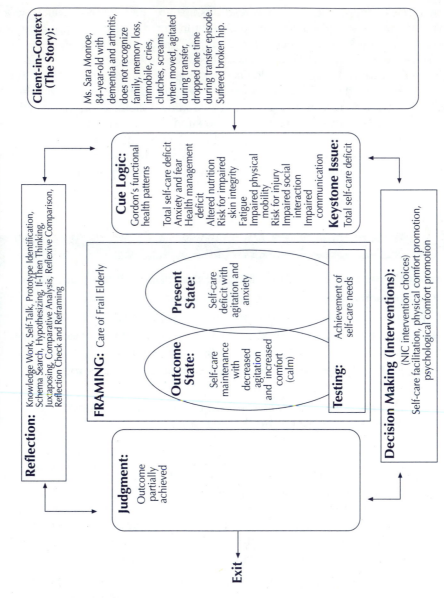

Reflection: Knowledge Work, Self-Talk, Prototype Identification, Schema Search, Hypothesizing, If-Then Thinking, Juxtaposing, Comparative Analysis, Reflexive Comparison, Reflection Check and Reframing

Client-in-Context (The Story):

Ms. Sara Monroe, 84-year-old with dementia and arthritis, does not recognize family, memory loss, immobile, cries, clutches, screams when moved, agitated during transfer, dropped one time during transfer episode. Suffered broken hip.

Cue Logic:
Gordon's functional health patterns

Total self-care deficit
Anxiety and fear
Health management deficit
Altered nutrition
Risk for impaired skin integrity
Fatigue
Impaired physical mobility
Risk for injury
Impaired social interaction
Impaired communication

Keystone Issue: Total self-care deficit

FRAMING: Care of Frail Elderly

Outcome State:
Self-care maintenance with decreased agitation and increased comfort (calm)

Present State:
Self-care deficit with agitation and anxiety

Testing: Achievement of self-care needs

Decision Making (Interventions):
(NIC intervention choices)
Self-care facilitation, physical comfort promotion, psychological comfort promotion

Judgment:
Outcome partially achieved

Exit

FIGURE 10-4 Completed OPT Model Worksheet for Ms. Sara Monroe

Juxtaposing

The side-by-side contrast of one state with the other suggests the gaps that need to be filled in order to achieve the outcome. The difference or gap evident between the present and desired state help create a test. The nurse contrasts self-care deficit with agitation and anxiety with a desired outcome of a self-care maintenance with an increase in comfort. The side-by-side comparison of these two states or conditions creates a gap. The gap must be bridged. Bridging the gap is influenced by clinical decisions and nursing actions. In order to achieve the desired outcome the nurse works with Ms. Monroe to decrease anxiety and agitation and increase self-care to the best of Ms. Monroe's abilities.

STOP AND THINK

1. **What evidence would you use to know the gap has been filled?**
2. **What nursing care actions or clinical decisions need to be made to obtain the evidence?**
3. **How will information contained in the Gordon, NANDA, and NIC nursing knowledge classification systems be useful as one reasons and reflects on this case?**

In Ms. Monroe's case, criteria for the test need to be established before the test can be conducted. What evidence will the nurse use to determine that the outcome of self-care maintained with comfort and calm was achieved? Obviously, a decrease in verbalization of agitated and anxious behavior would be one criterion to use. The self-care management would be evaluated by assessing the degree to which toileting, bathing, feeding, positioning, and grooming were accomplished by Ms. Monroe or nursing care personnel.

Decision Making (Interventions)

How is the nurse going to assist Ms. Monroe in moving from present state to outcome state? The goal of decision making is to select the interventions and actions that will have the most influence on the outcome and eliminate interventions and actions that have little or no influence on the outcome. NIC provides the knowledge required for decision making. For example, one of the decisions the nurse can make is to implement the intervention of self-care facilitation. Self-care facilitation is the category that contains interventions to provide or assist with routine activities of daily living (McCloskey & Bulechek, 1996). Specific interventions in this category are self-care assistance in bathing, hygiene, feeding, toileting, and grooming. Other clinical decisions or interventions the nurse might use to facilitate transition from present state to outcome state include physical comfort promotion (pain management), psychological comfort promotion (calming techniques), risk management (fall prevention), and behavior therapy (behavior modification). How will the nurses know if the clinical decisions she has made are working? She will know because of comparative analysis and application of the reflexive comparison thinking strategy. Reflexive comparison is a thinking strategy that involves constant comparison of the client's state from time of observation to time of observation.

Reflexive Comparison

Next time the nurse comes to see Ms. Monroe, the nurse will compare her progress with the nurse's last observation or visit. In this way, the nurse is using both the identified outcome criteria and Ms. Monroe as her own standard of progress or outcome achievement. By juxtaposing the outcome state criteria with a reflexive comparison of Ms. Monroe's current state, the nurse will have data and evidence that she can use in making a clinical judgment. For example, if Ms. Monroe achieved the outcome criteria of comfort and calm during self-care activities the outcome would have been achieved. If Ms. Monroe's condition deteriorates, however, reflection and reframing of keystone issues or the present state would need to take place. This situation would change the story and activate cue logic, resulting in the development of a different outcome state, present state, and test. Finally, Ms. Monroe could improve but not achieve or meet the desired outcome. If this were the case, then reflection about this is likely to provide new data and insights resulting in another set of clinical decisions or interventions to promote the transition to the outcome state. Data or evidence derived from these comparisons are the facts one uses to make clinical judgments.

For example, in Ms. Monroe's case, if she continues to yell, "Please don't let me fall" during transfer episodes, how would you use this evidence in making judgments about the achievement of the outcome? A test and reflexive comparison would continue until some progress was made toward self-care facilitation, physical comfort promotion, and psychological comfort promotion as well as behavioral management. Reflection and reasoning is likely to result in another OPT analysis and set of clinical decisions and clinical judgments.

STOP AND THINK

1. **Given Ms. Monroe's reaction, what judgments do you make about outcome achievement?**
2. **Based on Ms. Monroe's reaction, how would you reframe the situation? What do you think the desired outcome state is?**
3. **How did the OPT model help structure the reasoning in this case?**
4. **Do you think it is necessary to reframe the issues that need attention in Ms. Monroe's case?**

Reframing

Reframing is the thinking strategy of attributing a different meaning to the content or context of a situation given a set of cues, tests, decisions, or judgments. If different issues emerged or are not resolved, then reflection and decision making activates cue logic to identify new keystone issues that need attention. For example, perhaps fear is the real keystone issue in Ms. Monroe's story. Another issue is how long she will be able to maintain any self-care given her limitations. How might pain influence future self-care resource and deficits?

Reflection Check

A reflection check pinpoints what has been done correctly; it also identifies errors and provides insights and opportunities to identify and understand how to fix errors or reframe issues. Consider the following "Stop and Think."

STOP AND THINK

1. **If you were Ms. Monroe's nurse how would you reason differently about her story? Explain how past clinical experiences would influence your reasoning about this case.**

2. **Given this case, describe instances of your own use of self-talk, schema search, prototype identification, hypothesizing, if–then thinking, comparative analysis, juxtaposing, reflexive comparison, reframing, and reflection checking.**

3. **How will experience with this case influence future clinical reasoning if you encounter a client with a similar story?**

Use the Thinking Strategies Worksheet in Table 10-2 to identify specific examples from Ms. Monroe's case that illustrate your understanding and application of the thinking strategies.

SUMMARY

In this chapter knowledge and skills nurses need to practice and care for elderly clients were presented. Context-relevant diagnoses most often associated with long-term care clients were identified. The story of Ms. Sara Monroe, an 84-year-old client with dementia who experiences anxiety and agitation during her daily self-care routines was described. A Clinical Reasoning Web and OPT Model Worksheet were developed. Thinking strategies that support clinical reasoning were discussed. At the end of the chapter, readers had an opportunity to reflect and reframe some of the issues in Ms. Monroe's case and use the OPT model to structure clinical reasoning.

TABLE 10-2 Thinking Strategies Worksheet for Ms. Sara Monroe		
THINKING STRATEGY	**DEFINITION**	**EXAMPLE FROM MS. SARA MONROE'S CASE**
Knowledge Work	Active use of reading, memorizing, drilling, writing, reviewing research, and practicing to learn clinical vocabulary	
Self-Talk	Expressing one's thoughts to one's self	
Schema Search	Accessing general and/or specific patterns of past experiences that might apply to the current situation	
Prototype Identification	Using a model case as a reference point for comparative analysis	
Hypothesizing	Determining an explanation that that accounts for a set of facts can be tested by further investigation	
If–Then Thinking	Linking ideas and consequences together in a logical sequence	
Comparative Analysis	Considering the strengths and weaknesses of competing alternatives	
Juxtaposing	Putting the present-state condition next to the outcome state in a side-by-side contrast	
Reflexive Comparison	Constantly comparing the client's state from time of observation to time of observation	
Reframing	Attributing a different meaning to the content or context of a situation based on tests, decisions, or judgments	
Reflection Check	Self-examination and self-correction of critical thinking skills and thinking strategies that support clinical reasoning	

KEY CONCEPTS

1. Nurses who practice in long-term care settings need special knowledge and skills that involve understanding the unique needs of gerontological clients.

2. Clinical reasoning about client needs in long-term care draws on several knowledge classification systems.

3. The structure of clinical reasoning in long-term care is similar to reasoning challenges in other contexts.

4. The thinking strategies of self-talk, schema search, prototype identification, hypothesizing, if–then thinking, comparative analysis, juxtaposing, reflexive comparison, reframing, and reflection check support clinical reasoning.

STUDY QUESTIONS AND ACTIVITIES

1. If you were 78 years old and in good health, but could not maintain an independent living situation any longer, what kind of long-term care facility would you consider? What criteria would be important to you? What qualities would you look for in the staff and environment of such a facility?

2. Identify a long-term care facility in your community. Find out the profile of the residents. Based on this information, what nursing diagnoses can you predict are the most prevalent in that setting?

3. The focus of this chapter was on the elderly in long-term care. However, some residents in these facilities can be young, such as a middle-aged person who has a stroke. How does the age of the client influence your thinking, reasoning, and care planning?

4. If money were not an object, what kind of long-term care facility could you design? Develop a scenario that describes a long-term care facility in the year 2020.

REFERENCES

American Nurses Association. (1995). *Scope and standards of gerontological nursing practice.* Washington, DC: American Nurses Publishing.

Bahr, S. (1994). Overview of gerontological nursing. In M. Hogstel (Ed.), *Nursing care of the older adult* (Chapter 1). New York: John Wiley & Sons.

Lekan-Rutledge, D. (1997). Gerontological nursing in long-term care facilities. In M. Matteson, E. McConnell, & A. Linton (Eds.), *Gerontological nursing concepts and practices* (2nd ed., pp. 931–965). Philadelphia, PA: W. B. Saunders.

Matteson, M., McConnell, E., & Linton, A. (Eds.). (1997). *Gerontological nursing concepts and practices* (2nd ed.). Philadelphia, PA: W. B. Saunders.

McCloskey, J., & Bulechek, G. (1996). *Nursing interventions classification* (2nd ed.) St. Louis, MO: Mosby.

Mezey, M., Lynaugh, J., & Cartier, M. (1989). Re-ordering values: The teaching nursing home program. In Mezey, M., Lynaugh, J., and Cartier, M. (Eds.), *Nursing homes and nursing care: Lessons from the teaching nursing homes* (4). New York: Springer.

Puzicka, S. (1997). Nursing diagnoses influenced by setting of care. In M. Matteson, E. McConnell, & A. Linton. (Eds.). (1997). *Gerontological nursing concepts and practices* (2nd ed., pp. 829–853). Philadelphia, PA: W. B. Saunders.

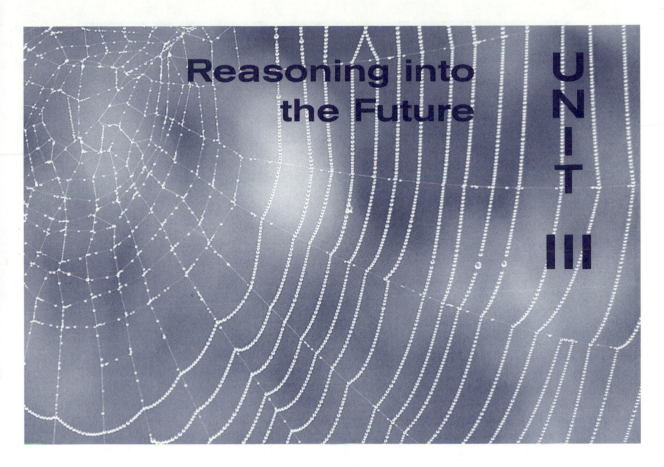

Reasoning into the Future

UNIT III

Unit III contains three chapters. The use of the OPT model to facilitate clinical supervision and development of therapeutic competence is discussed in Chapter 11. The concepts of academic, practical, successful, and nursing intelligence are defined. Clinical supervision helps clinicians develop successful nursing intelligence. In Chapter 12, use of the OPT model for the development of middle-range theories for nursing practice is described. Using current nursing knowledge classification systems, one can use the structure of the OPT model to organize thinking and reasoning about relevant middle-range theories. Finally, in Chapter 13, future health care trends and the consequences of these trends for clinical reasoning are noted. The contributions of the OPT model for practice, education, and research in nursing are noted as the profession moves toward the development and testing of theories for clinical reasoning.

CHAPTER 11

Using the OPT Model to Support Clinical Supervision

COMPETENCIES

After completing this chapter, the reader should be able to:

1. Discuss and define academic, practical, successful, and nursing intelligence.
2. Discuss the concept and purposes of clinical supervision.
3. Explain how the OPT model can be used to structure and organize the clinical supervision process.
4. Discuss a set of questions that facilitate the supervision process.

INTRODUCTION

As health care systems are restructured and redesigned, nurses are going to find themselves supervising ancillary health care workers. Helping others reason about complex care situations is not an easy job. Nurses need to develop clinical supervision skills. The art and science of clinical reasoning are foundations for the clinical supervisory process. The purpose of this chapter is to discuss the different kinds of intelligence that are needed to be successful in professional practice environments. Academic, practical, successful, and nursing intelligence are defined and discussed. These intelligences are essential aspects of the clinical supervisory process. The OPT model is proposed as one way to think about and structure clinical supervision sessions. With the OPT model in mind, it is easy to lead people through a systematic analysis of keystone issues and desired outcomes in a particular case. The structure and process of the OPT model helps develop the multiple intelligences one needs to be successful. Other tools such as the Clinical Reasoning Web, OPT Model Worksheet, and Thinking Strategies Worksheet help organize thinking and reasoning about complex situations that demand supervisory attention.

ACADEMIC, PRACTICAL, SUCCESSFUL, AND NURSING INTELLIGENCE

Nurses need academic, practical, successful, and nursing intelligence to deliver and provide quality care. Sternberg (1996) observes that intelligence is the ability to cope with demands created by novel situations and problems. Intelligence is the application of experience. Use of reasoning and inference as a guide is considered intelligence.

Sternberg (1985; 1988; 1996) makes a distinction among academic, practical, and successful intelligence. Academic intelligence is measured by IQ tests; it is knowledge focused on what "should" work. Academic problems are well defined, are formulated by others, and usually come with all the information that is necessary for problem solution. Generally, academic problems have only one correct answer and method for obtaining that answer. Often academic problems are unrelated to everyday experience.

In contrast, practical intelligence is the ability to apply mental abilities to everyday situations. Practical intelligence involves learning to manage oneself, others, and tasks. The "street smarts" of practical intelligence are tacit and embedded in experience. Sternberg (1988) notes that practical problems differ from academic problems in five ways. First, practical problems are not well defined and are not formulated by others. Second, one often does not have all the information needed to solve the problem. Third, there is rarely a single solution to practical problems. Fourth, everyday experience can be used to solve practical problems. Finally, practical intelligence is knowledge focused on what does work.

For example, consider Benner's (1984) work. By talking with nurses she "discovered" and made explicit the tacit knowledge or practical intelligences involved in the reality of nursing practice. Benner identified the following practical domains of nursing:

- the helping role
- the teaching-coaching function
- the diagnostic and client monitoring function
- the effective management of rapidly changing situations domain
- the administration and monitoring of therapeutic interventions and regimens

- the monitoring and ensuring the quality of health care practices
- the domain of organizational and work role competencies

Benner (1984) makes a distinction between "knowing that" and "knowing how." She suggests that practical knowledge may elude scientific formulations. She also believes that knowledge development in an applied discipline consists of extending practical "know-how" through theory-based scientific investigations and through sharing the existent "know-how" developed through clinical experience.

Practical experiences (clinical dialogue) combined with academic experiences (theory) build nursing knowledge and enhance individual and collective nursing intelligence. The nursing intelligence quotient (NIQ) is a function of academic and practical intelligence modified by reflection-in-action. It is an ability to cope with demands created by novel nursing situations or new nursing problems. NIQ is the ability to apply what is learned from nursing care experiences and to use reasoning and inference effectively as a guide for the development of nursing care knowledge. NIQ is a function of knowing that, knowing how, and knowing why. NIQ is a function of a clinician's ability to maintain curiosity and a sense of surprise in her or his work. NIQ is enhanced every time nurses talk with themselves and others in a reflective way about client care situations. The common dominator of NIQ is reflection-in-action.

Reflection-in-action is a term used by Schon (1983) to describe the process by which professionals think and act. Reflection-in-action is the ability to consciously talk with your self and others about a practice situation. The OPT model thinking strategies of self-talk, prototype identification, schema search, hypothesizing, if–then thinking, comparative analysis, juxtaposing, reflexive comparison, reframing, and reflective check are the specific techniques of reflection-in-action.

Reflective skills are central to the "art" by which practitioners deal with uncertain, unique situations. When individuals reflect-in-action they become scientist-scholars in the practice context. As scientist-scholars they are concerned about what works, but are also curious about what does not work. What doesn't work helps pinpoint the next target for inquiry.

Each clinical case, scenario, and vignette we encounter provides an opportunity for reflection-in-action. Clinical supervision is an opportunity to help peers, colleagues, and subordinates reflect in order to develop prerequisite skills and the spirit of inquiry essential for professional practice.

STOP AND THINK

1. **How can clinical supervision help develop the knowledge, intent, reflection, curiosity, tolerance for ambiguity, self-confidence, and professional motivation necessary for clinical reasoning?**

CLINICAL SUPERVISION AND THE DEVELOPMENT OF SUCCESSFUL INTELLIGENCE

The purpose of clinical supervision is to promote an individual's success and therapeutic competence. Clinical supervision is an interpersonal process that helps people identify strengths, know weaknesses, capitalize on assets, compensate for or correct weaknesses, and contribute to their success. Loganbill, Hardy, and Delworth (1982) define supervision as an intensive, interpersonally focused, one-to-one relationship in which one person is designated to facilitate the therapeutic competence in the other person. Webb (1997) notes that clinical supervision serves a number of purposes. First, it establishes a formal system for practitioners to explore, discover, and examine their practice in a safe and supportive environment. Second, clinical supervision allows individuals to develop their thoughts and actions in a way that leads to enhanced care delivery to the patient or client group. Third, clinical supervision enables practitioners to accept accountability for their own practice and development. Finally, clinical supervision serves the purpose of containing the stresses of working in a demanding environment within the workplace.

Clinical supervision enables people to learn, develop, and reflect on practice problems and gain insight, support, and guidance that enhances care and professional development (Pesut & Williams, 1990). Active use of clinical supervision is one way to sustain lifelong learning. Remember, this competence was deemed an essential one for health care providers for the future (Shugars, O'Neil, & Bader, 1991).

STOP AND THINK

1. **What are your images, impressions, and associations concerning the term "clinical supervision"?**
2. **Think of a clinical supervisor you admire. What qualities or characteristics make this person admirable?**
3. **How has clinical supervision contributed to your personal or professional development?**

Through the process of clinical supervision, one develops nursing intelligence and successful intelligence. Sternberg (1996) defines and outlines what comprises successful intelligence:

1. Successfully intelligent people don't wait for problems to hit them over the head. They recognize their existence before they get out of hand and begin the process of solving them.

2. Successfully intelligent people define problems correctly and thereby solve those problems that really confront them, rather than extraneous ones. In this way, the same problems don't keep coming back into their lives. They also make the effort to decide which problems are worth solving and which are not.

3. Successfully intelligent people carefully formulate strategies for problem solving. In particular, they focus on long-range planning rather than rushing in and later having to rethink their strategies.

4. Successfully intelligent people represent information about a problem as accurately as possible, with a focus on how they can use that information effectively.

5. Successfully intelligent people think carefully about allocating resources for both the short and long term. They consider risk–reward ratios and then choose the allocations they believe will maximize their return.

6. Successfully intelligent people do not always make the correct decisions, but they monitor and evaluate their decisions and then correct their errors as they discover them.

STOP AND THINK

1. **As you review the characteristics of successfully intelligent people in regard to problem solving, where are your own strengths?**

2. **What developmental needs or areas for improvement can you identify that will maximize your successful intelligence?**

3. **Given the context of clinical supervision, how does one foster successful intelligence if one is the supervisor?**

4. **Given the context of clinical supervision, how does one foster successful intelligence if one is the supervisee?**

Whether one is giving or receiving supervision, the supervisory process starts with a story. Sharing the elements of the story helps contextualize and frame the issues, problems, and dilemmas that need to be resolved. We believe the OPT model is one way to think about structuring the supervisory process. The structure and parts of the model lend themselves to all of the elements involved in a supervisory session. Stories lead to framing some issue in terms of the present state. Often the main contribution of a supervisor is to help the supervisee determine an outcome. Additionally, clinical decisions and choices of action help resolve situations based on evidence and judgments of outcome achievement. Supervisors help supervisees reflect, reason, and reframe facts when necessary.

USING OPT FOR CLINICAL SUPERVISION.

Thus far we have used the OPT model to help structure the reasoning about client cases. To this point we have used nursing knowledge classification systems for the clinical reasoning content. Consider now how the OPT model in Figure 11-1 can assist you in structuring a clinical supervision session. The elements and questions that support clinical supervision are contained within the model. We believe using the OPT model to structure thinking and reasoning in clinical supervision sessions will assist individuals in considering many of the elements of successful, academic, practical, and nursing intelligence associated with clinical reasoning.

Since the word "supervision" means literally to "oversee," a supervisor oversees the work of another with the responsibility for the quality of that work (Leddick & Bernand, 1980). The OPT model is a useful way to think about and organize the oversight of a supervisee's thinking.

Students are most familiar with educational clinical supervision. These supervision experiences help students learn about nursing interventions used in patient care. As students mature they develop confidence and expertise. However, new situations emerge and one may not have the experience to reason effectively about the situation. In these cases it is wise to seek clinical supervision.

Clinical supervision is one mechanism to enhance nursing intelligence since clinical supervision involves reflection-on-action. Reflection is increased by talking with each other about situations encountered, responses observed, and care solutions that are

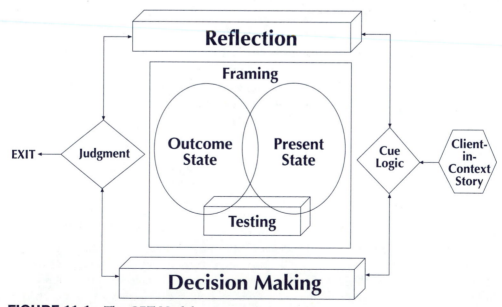

FIGURE 11-1 The OPT Model

effective. Case studies, client care conferences, formal and informal consultations, and use of clinical exemplars or critical incidents increase reflection and dialogue among students and practitioners. Discussion of how cases are alike and how they are different is another way to encourage reflection and build clinical knowledge. The OPT model coupled with the thinking strategies provides the structure and techniques for helping people think through complex situations.

Clinical supervision is accomplished through a dialogue and set of questions that parallel the structure of the OPT model. In Box 11-1 are several questions supervisors can use to help supervisees reason about specific situations with the OPT model structure as a framework.

BOX 11-1 Questions That Support OPT Model Use in Supervision

1. Tell me the story.
2. What are you thinking about the client situation?
3. What diagnoses have you generated as a result of your thinking?
4. What evidence supports those diagnoses?
5. Have you drawn a Clinical Reasoning Web to relate your ideas and thinking?
6. As you consider the whole story, are there themes that emerge?
7. How are you framing this situation? What assumptions have you made?
8. How have you defined the present state?
9. What is the desired outcome?
10. What is the gap between the outcome and the present state?
11. What evidence will fill the gap?
12. How will you know the outcome is achieved?
13. What clinical decisions or interventions are you going to make to help move the client from the present to the desired state?
14. How and why are you considering these choices? What are the risks and benefits, short-term and long-term gains for each?
15. Are these decisions and choices within your span of control? If they involve others, how will you negotiate participation and action?
16. Have you had experiences similar to this before? If so, what was successful then? Do you think it can be applied in this situation?
17. In my experience, I would frame this situation this way. How does this frame change, modify, or influence your thinking?
18. What is your clinical judgment at this point?
19. What do you plan to do next?
20. How can I help you further?

Most clinical supervision sessions begin with the discussion of a client's story. One of the key elements of a supervisory relationship is to help the employee reflect on the cue logic associated with the story. In fact, each part of the OPT model can become the focus for a set of questions that encourage reflection. Asking employees how, specifically, they are thinking about each element enables the clinical supervisor to uncover hidden assumptions, values, beliefs, and ideas and hold them up for explicit analysis and understanding. Sometimes a clinical supervisor helps frame problems and issues in a new way. Once a frame is established, outcomes are evident. Juxtaposing or making explicit the side-by-side comparison of specified outcome state criteria with present-state data is also a clinical supervision opportunity. This juxtaposition creates a gap analysis and thus the conditions for a test. Since the goal of care management is bridging the gap between present state and desired outcome state, supervisors help employees make clinical decisions.

Decision making is supported through the use and application of schema searches, prototype identification, and comparative analysis. The process of considering the strengths and weaknesses of competing alternatives is supported by if–then thinking and hypothesizing. Supervisors can explicitly ask questions that help employees recall facts and knowledge, think about prototypes, access schemas, and use if–then thinking, comparative analysis, and reflexive comparison in a systematic way. For example, a supervision question such as "What are the facts?" or "Have you had an experience like this one before?" facilitates recall and schema search. "What will happen if . . . ?" is a question that is likely to activate hypothesis generation and if–then thinking. "What were the baseline data associated with the client's condition?" is a question that activates the thinking strategies of comparative analysis and reflexive comparison.

Clinical judgments are critical. Supervision questions that help thinking in this process are "Have you achieved your desired result?" " What is missing based on your desired outcome criteria?" "Is there another explanation, frame, or way of looking at the problem that would account for the facts at hand?" Certainly other questions will arise during the course of the clinical supervision dialogue.

The OPT model structures the clinical supervision process by organizing the elements of the story, frame, present state–outcome state, test, and judgment. The astute clinical supervisor knows what thinking strategies support clinical reasoning. Use of a Clinical Reasoning Web and OPT Model Worksheet help make the thinking strategies explicit and relevant to the specific case under consideration. Fundamentally supervision is a learning process. It is important that employees perceive supervisors as role models. Use of the OPT tools and techniques is bound to increase the effectiveness and efficiency of the clinical supervision process. The outcomes of such effectiveness will be an increase in the academic, practical, nursing, and successful intelligence that is a part of professional nursing practice. Figure 11-2 shows a blank OPT Model Worksheet. How might you use this structure to guide your thinking and interactions with the people whom you supervise?

OPT Model Worksheet

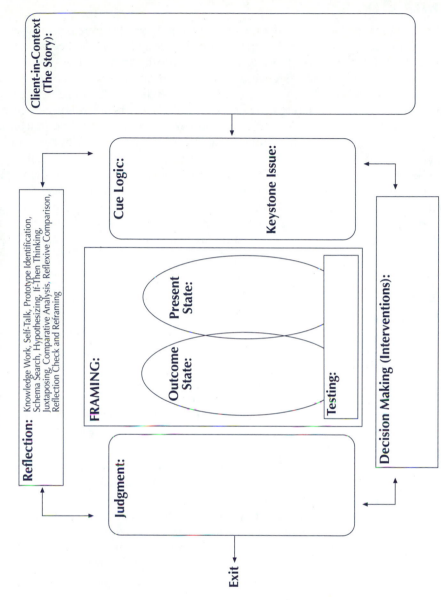

FIGURE 11-2 OPT Model Worksheet: Structure for the Supervision Process

SUMMARY

Academic intelligence is insufficient for successful performance in real-world settings. Successful and practical intelligence are also needed. Nursing intelligence was defined as a function of a clinician's ability to maintain curiosity and a sense of surprise in his or her work. Nursing intelligence develops when one appreciates strengths and recognizes barriers in understandings, skills, and abilities. Nursing intelligence is enhanced through clinical supervision and when practitioners talk among themselves and make implicit knowledge explicit. Nursing intelligence grows when practitioner-scholars identify and discuss the multiple intelligences that exist in nursing and use insights gained to develop the practical and academic knowledge that is nursing science. Use of the OPT model can help guide clinical supervision because the thinking strategies of the model are the techniques for reflection and clinical reasoning. OPT encourages the use and application of the analytic, creative, practical, and successful intelligences that contribute to professional practice. Supervisors play a critical role in asking questions that stimulate reflection and the activation of the many thinking strategies that support clinical reasoning.

KEY CONCEPTS

1. Clinical supervision is both an art and science. As health care contexts experience restructuring and redesign, nurses are going to find themselves supervising a variety of ancillary health care workers. Clinical supervision is a skill that must be developed.

2. Supervision is an intensive, interpersonally focused, one-to-one relationship in which one person is designated to facilitate therapeutic competence in the other person. The word "supervision" means literally to "oversee." Thus a supervisor is one who oversees the work of another with the responsibility for the quality of that work.

3. Clinical supervision establishes formal systems for practitioners to explore, discover, and examine their practice in a safe and supportive environment. Clinical supervision allows individuals to develop their thoughts and actions in a way that leads to enhanced care delivery to the patient or client group. Clinical supervision enables practitioners to accept accountability for their own practice and development. Clinical supervision serves the purpose of containing the stresses of working in a demanding environment within the workplace.

4. The OPT model can become the structure for guiding questions that encourage reflection. Asking employees how they are thinking about each element of the OPT model enables the clinical supervisor to uncover hidden assumptions, values, beliefs, and ideas and hold them up for explicit analysis and understanding.

5. The essence of clinical supervision is the conscious activation on the part of the supervisor to help the supervisee use the thinking strategies that support clinical reasoning.

STUDY QUESTIONS AND ACTIVITIES

1. What are the essential elements of clinical supervision in your mind? Write your own definition of clinical supervision and discuss it with a peer or colleague.

2. Develop a plan for how you will gain skill as a clinical supervisor.

3. Based on the OPT model, develop a set of supervision questions that could be put on a card in your pocket. Make sure the questions raise the key issues for reflecting on clinical situations to achieve desired outcomes.

4. How is supervision of ancillary nursing personnel different from supervision with a peer or colleague? Can you adapt the OPT model to accommodate these differences?

5. What are some of the ethical and legal consequences of clinical supervision?

6. How might adherence to the OPT model be useful as you consider the ethical and legal issues associated with clinical supervision?

REFERENCES

Benner, P. (1984). *From novice to expert: Power and excellence in nursing practice.* Menlo Park, CA: Addison-Wesley.

Leddick, G., & Bernard, J. (1980). The history of supervision: A critical review. *Counselor Education and Supervision, 19,* 186–196.

Loganbill, C., Hardy, E., & Delworth, U. (1982). Supervision: A conceptual model. *Counseling Psychologist, 10*(1), 3–42.

Pesut, D., & Williams, C. (1990). The nature of clinical supervision in psychiatric nursing: A survey of clinical specialists. *Archives of Psychiatric Nursing, 4*(3), 188–194.

Schon, D. (1983). *The reflective practitioner.* New York: Basic Books.

Shugars, D. A., O'Neil, E. H., & Bader, J. D. (Eds.). (1991). *Healthy America: Practitioners for 2005, an agenda for action for U.S. health professional schools.* Durham, NC: The Pew Health Professions Commission.

Sternberg, R. (1996). *Successful intelligence.* New York: Simon & Schuster.

Sternberg, R. (1988). *The triarchic mind: A new theory of human intelligence.* New York: Viking.

Sternberg, R. (1985). Implicit theories of intelligence, creativity, and wisdom. *Journal of Personality and Social Psychology, 49,* 607–627.

Webb, B. (1997). Auditing a clinical supervision training program. *Nursing Standard, 11*(34), 34–49.

CHAPTER 12

Using the OPT Model for Middle Range Theory Development

COMPETENCIES

After completing this chapter, the reader should be able to:

1. Describe the importance of theory development and theory testing for nursing.

2. Explain four levels of inquiry related to practice theory.

3. Describe the importance of knowledge classification systems for theory development.

4. Consider how the OPT model combined with NANDA, NIC, and NOC organizes theories and knowledge for nursing practice.

5. Evaluate the potential of the OPT model for helping structure knowledge and develop middle-range theories for clinical practice.

INTRODUCTION

The OPT model helps structure clinical reasoning. The model is also useful as a guide and framework for clinical supervision. Another use of the OPT model is the organization of nursing knowledge into middle-range theories. Middle-range theories can be tested through research. In the first part of this chapter, the importance of theory development and theory testing activities for advancing the scientific basis for nursing practice is described. Four levels of inquiry related to the development of practice theory are reviewed. Because of the tremendous advances in the development of nursing knowledge, the profession is at the threshold of a new era. The OPT model, coupled with nursing knowledge content, is potentially useful for organizing diagnoses, interventions, and outcomes in a unique way. Organizing problems, outcomes, and interventions together enables clinicians to develop and test middle-range theories that have practice relevance.

PRACTICE, THEORY, AND SCIENCE

Nursing is a practice profession. Clinical experiences helps one see patterns of behaviors. Based on these patterns one knows what to do in certain situations. Clinical knowledge leads to practical intelligence (Sternberg, 1985). Practical intelligence is supported by analytic and creative intelligence, which helps develop science. The rules of science require the profession use knowledge that is valid, reliable, and evidence-based. As nursing knowledge is developed and classified, it needs to be organized in ways that make it useful. We believe the OPT model is a scaffold upon which nursing knowledge can be organized, developed, and tested through research studies.

INTEGRATING THEORY, PRACTICE, AND RESEARCH

Practice is the keystone of nursing. Students are eager to gain the practical intelligence that comes from working in the real world. Working with individuals, families, and communities is gratifying. Helping others is one of the attractions of the nursing profession. Students soon realize that real-world experience gained in clinical settings is influenced and supported by academic intelligence. Clinical experience provides the opportunities to apply what one knows and gain more knowledge in the process. Professional development requires attention to concepts, theories, and real-world experience. As one gains real-world experience, one realizes that sometimes concepts and theories do not explain experience encountered in the real world. Consider the questions in the following "STOP AND THINK" feature.

STOP AND THINK

1. Do you prefer learning theories and concepts first, and then applying them to clinical situations?

2. Do you prefer to have clinical experiences and then search out theories that help make sense of those experiences?

3. In your experience have concepts and theories helped explain what you have experienced in practice?

4. Are there situations you have experienced in practice that cannot be explained by concepts and theories?

5. When you experience this gap, what do you do?

6. Do you use research findings to support your thinking and practice?

As clinical experiences and learning accumulate, nurses organize this knowledge in broader generalizations. These broader generalizations become formal theories. Theory enables one to describe, explain, and predict behavior in the world. Students quickly realize there are many theories of and for nursing that help describe, explain, predict, and evaluate nursing care for people in need. The need for theory in nursing is linked with the need for research-based knowledge that guides practice. As the profession strives to develop a scientific base for practice, knowledge generated from research becomes a professional obligation and responsibility.

Practice informs theory and research, and theory and research inform and support practice. Fawcett (1995) uses the double-helix structure of DNA as a metaphor to illustrate these relationships. Practically speaking, some treat practice, research, and theory as separate and distinct knowledge categories. Such partitioning prevents professional development. Blegen and Tripp-Reimer (1997) describe and discuss the advantages and disadvantages of keeping these knowledge categories separate. Keeping categories separate has the advantage of allowing each category to become developed in its own right. However, when the categories are closely connected, new methods of conceptualizing, testing, and applying knowledge need to be developed and tested. The results of knowledge development efforts in the past 10 years has led us to another understanding about relationships among practice, theory, and research. The nursing profession has achieved a level of development whereby the profession can begin to build bridges among knowledge classification structures. The development and testing of middle-range theories is where this bridging takes place.

PRACTICE AND MIDDLE-RANGE THEORIES FOR NURSING

In the late 1960s two philosophers, Dickoff and James (1968), outlined the essential components of a practice theory for nursing. Diers (1979) used their ideas to develop a nursing research textbook. In this text, Diers used Dickoff and James' notions of different levels of practice theory to illustrate how traditional research methods support the development of practice theory associated with four levels of inquiry. The four levels of practice theory are: factor isolating or naming; factor relating situation depicting, or situation describing; situation relating or predictive; and situation producing or prescriptive. Following is a brief description of each of these levels. Each level is associated with a level of inquiry that becomes increasingly complex. The level of inquiry, kind of question, study design, kind of answer theory, and other names for study designs are outlined in Table 12-1.

TABLE 12-1   Levels of Inquiry Related to Levels of Practice Theory

LEVEL OF INQUIRY	KIND OF QUESTION	STUDY DESIGN	KIND OF ANSWER (THEORY)	OTHER NAMES FOR STUDY DESIGN
1	What is this?	Factor searching	Factor isolating (naming)	Exploratory Formulative Descriptive Situational Control
2	What's happening here?	Relation searching	Factor relating (situation depicting, situation describing)	Exploratory Descriptive
3	What will happen if . . . ?	Association testing Causal hypothesis testing	Situation relating (predictive)	Correlational Survey Design Nonexperimental Natural experiment Experimental Explanatory Predictive
4	How can I make . . . happen?	Prescription testing	Situation producing (prescriptive)	

Reprinted with permission. Diers, D. (1979). *Research in nursing practice.* Philadelphia, PA: Lippincott, p. 54.

Level 1 inquiry is called factor isolating or naming practice theory. At this level the question "What is this?" guides theory development activities. This level of practice theory involves describing and naming concepts so practitioners have conceptual labels, handles, or tools for describing what they see and experience in practice. For example, definitions of experience and patterns of observed behavior are identified. The creation and development of NANDA nursing diagnoses are a type of factor isolating, Level 1 inquiry in the quest to develop a practice theory. The development and classification of nursing interventions and outcomes are additional examples of factor isolating theory. Concept development or naming of experiences as well as concept analysis is important to factor isolating practice theory work (Morse, 1995). This type of theory development activity is supported by conventional research designs that are exploratory, descriptive, or formulative.

Level 2 inquiry is called factor relating, situation depicting, or situation describing practice theory. This theory is a logical consequence of factor isolation. Once concepts have been described and defined, people put the concepts to use and ask questions about how concepts are related. The second level of inquiry answers the question "What is happening here?" At this level curiosity and methods come together to connect and order concepts. For example, how is self-care related to symptom monitoring activities? Two concepts, self-care and symptom monitoring, are linked in hopes of explaining what is happening in practice. Relation searching, exploratory, or descriptive designs assist clinicians in answering questions about linkages among concepts. For example, what are the correlations among pain, anxiety, and comfort in regard to symptom management and self-care practices?

Level 3 inquiry is known as situation relating or predictive practice theory. At this level curious clinicians ask the question "What will happen if . . . ?" Research designs at this level are often correlational, survey, or nonexperimental studies. At this level, causal hypothesis testing begins to be developed. For example, do people who can self-administer pain medication use more or less pain medication than people who must rely on health care providers for pain medication administration? In this example one is trying to relate elements of the situation in hopes of some prediction and association among ideas, concepts, or hypotheses. Use of naturalistic studies, experimental, explanatory or predictive research designs are means to answer the "What will happen . . . if" question.

Level 4 inquiry is known as producing or prescriptive practice theory. At this level one hopes to answer the question, "How can I make . . . happen?" In other words, how can the nurse use knowledge and theory to achieve a desired outcome or produce a specific situation? How is it that nurses can prescribe interventions in order to achieve desired outcomes? Situation producing or prescriptive theory contains prescriptions for activities to bring about goals defined within the theory. Well-developed prescriptions meet the following survey list or set of criteria established by Dickoff and James (1968). The survey list includes information about six elements:

- who or what performs the activity
- who receives the activity
- what context the activity is performed in
- details about the procedure or how it is done
- why it is done
- what end result is desired

The survey list is a fundamental part of the prescriptive theory for practice.

The four levels of inquiry are the building blocks for theory development and testing as nursing tries to develop a science base for prescriptive nursing practice.

STOP AND THINK

1. **What do you think are the relationships among theory, practice, and research?**
2. **Do you like the way Diers organized the different levels of inquiry and types of theory?**
3. **When you studied research and nursing theory, did you discuss how practice theory is different from pure research?**
4. **Can you see why the work of NANDA could be described as factor isolating or naming theory development?**
5. **Once factors are named and described, they can be related to other factors to help describe and explain situations. What, for example, do you think the relationships are between immobility and impaired skin integrity? Can you create a mini theory about these relationships? How do they influence and relate to each other? How could such a theory and interventions be tested?**
6. **Given the results of evidence derived from the research conducted in question 5, how is possible to develop a middle-range theory about the effects of immobility on skin integrity? To what degree would such a theory be useful in practice?**
7. **Do you consider yourself a middle-range theorist?**

Today it is much easier to develop practice theories because of the factor isolating and naming work that has gone on in the past 10 years. Specifically, the work of NANDA, NIC, and NOC is a tremendous contribution to the naming, categorizing, and classifying of nursing knowledge. The next few decades are likely to see a burst of theory development activities that will use the work of these organizations. With the foundation of these knowledge classification systems, people are now able to use nursing terms to spin and weave middle-range theories that have practice relevance. Such middle-range theory development activities have research consequences and educational implications. Middle-range theory development is something you do all the time as you think about relationships among ideas and how to make the most of your nursing care actions.

MIDDLE-RANGE THEORY DEVELOPMENT

The nursing profession's fascination with grand theories was a professional developmental stage necessary for the profession's legitimization as an academic discipline (Suppe, 1994). Now that nursing is accepted in academic circles, the next stage of development is a focus on development of middle-range theories. Middle-range theories, as opposed to grand theories, deal with practice-relevant issues. Middle-range theories seek to describe, explain, predict, and prescribe nursing actions and consequences related to a selected focus. These theories are comprised of working hypotheses essential to research. Middle-range theories are abstract yet rely on facts and empirical data so questions can be asked about interventions for practice (Chinn, 1994). As the name implies, middle-range theories address concepts toward a middle scope of interest (Blegen & Tripp-Reimer, 1997). The key components of a middle-range theory are three or more concepts linked together with logical propositions that can be tested (Walker & Avant, 1995). For example, one could have middle-range theory about the relationship among patient-controlled analgesia and anxiety. A proposition that could be tested might be something like: the more patients control the analgesia, the less postoperative anxiety they will have in regard to pain. In this example one is linking the concepts of patient-controlled analgesia, anxiety, and pain management together. Can you think of a way to conduct research on this theory? The primary function of theory is to explain and predict one phenomenon on the basis of knowledge of another phenomena. Other recent examples of middle-range theories are symptom management (Lenz, Pugh, Mulligan, Gift, & Suppe, 1997), resilience (Polk, 1997), nurse-expressed empathy (Olson & Hanchett, 1997), and chronotherapeutic interventions for postsurgical pain (Auvil-Novak, 1997). We suggest that the OPT model can be used to structure middle-range theory.

USING OPT TO STRUCTURE MIDDLE-RANGE THEORY

The knowledge contained in the classification systems of NANDA, NIC, and NOC can be used to build middle-range theories. The structure of the OPT model is like a blueprint or scaffold (See Figure 12-1.) that can be used to link information from the three taxonomies together. Such middle-range theory development has been proposed by Blegen and Tripp-Reimer (1997).

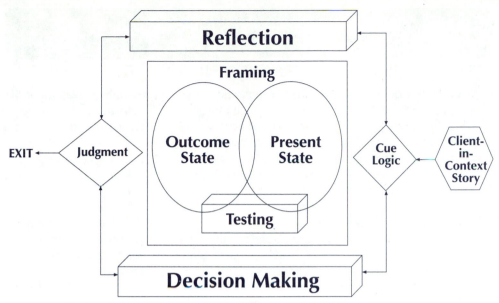

FIGURE 12-1 The OPT Model

Consider how one might use the OPT model with information about the diagnosis of activity intolerance and the nursing interventions and outcomes identified in Table 12-2. Consider how this data can be translated into propositions, using the structure of the OPT model. Think about relationships among the diagnosis of activity intolerance and the outcome of ambulation with balance. Now look at the clinical decisions or nursing action choices from the NIC column that the nurse must decide on. How does energy management influence ambulation with balance? Might you develop a middle-range theory about these factors that can be tested?

For the client with a diagnosis or present state of activity intolerance, a desired outcome might be "walks effectively." Clinical decisions or NIC interventions such as energy management and range of motion exercise are used to transition the client from the present state of activity intolerance to effective walking. A middle-range theory tests the relationship of propositions that range of motion exercises facilitate energy management by building strength and endurance to foster effective walking, resulting in a decrease in activity intolerance.

What might a prescriptive nursing practice theory for this look like? One can develop and create situation-producing theories using a survey list: Agency—who or what performs the activity? Client—who receives the activity? What framework is necessary in what specific context? How specifically is the procedure accomplished? What are the end results? Using this survey list and examples of energy management, the nurse can prescribe who does range of motion, with whom, where, when, how, and with what expected increase in joint function and mobility. Such a theory can be translated

TABLE 12-2 Linking NANDA Diagnoses with NIC Interventions and NOC Outcomes

DIAGNOSIS—NANDA	INTERVENTION—NIC	OUTCOME—NOC
Activity intolerance: A state in which an individual has insufficient physiological or psychological energy to endure or complete required or desired daily activities	1. Body mechanics promotion: Facilitating the use of posture and movement in daily activities to prevent fatigue and musculoskeletal strain and injury	Ambulating: Walking indicators
Defining characteristics	Activities	Walks with effective gait
Verbal report of fatigue or weakness	Collaborate with physical therapist in planning	Walks up and down stairs
Abnormal heart rate or blood pressure in response to activity	Instruct on structure and function	Walks moderate distances
Exertional discomfort or dyspnea	Monitor improvement in client's posture and body mechanics	Mobility level indicators
EKG changes indicating arrhythmias or ischemia	2. Energy management: Regulating energy use to treat or prevent fatigue and optimize function	Balance performance
	Activities	Joint movement
	Determine client's physical limitations	Muscle function
	Determine what and how much activity is required to build endurance	
	Monitor response to exercise	
	Encourage alternate rest and exercise	
	Use passive and active range of motion	

Tables reprinted with permission from Blegen, M., & Tripp-Reimer, T. (1997). Implications of nursing taxonomies for middle-range theory development. *Advances in Nursing Science,* *19*(3), 37–49.

STOP AND THINK

1. **Think of a client for whom you provided care that had a nursing diagnosis of activity intolerance.**
2. **Review the NIC interventions in Table 12-2. Which of these interventions did you use with this client?**
3. **What was your goal or desired outcome for your client? Was it ambulating with an effective gait? Mobility with balance? On a five-point scale, how might you rate outcome achievement?**
4. **How is energy management and range of motion exercise related to your outcome and resolution of the nursing diagnosis?**
5. **Based on your experiences, can you think about relationships among these concepts that would become a middle-range theory associated with energy management, mobility, and activity intolerance?**
6. **How might one continue to develop these ideas?**
7. **What level of practice theory would this be?**
8. **Could you foresee developing a prescriptive nursing practice theory that helps describe, explain, and predict nursing care issues associated with activity intolerance, exercise, and mobility?**

into a research project from which evidence can be derived in order to make a judgment about the effectiveness of the theory.

THINKING STRATEGIES

The thinking strategies that support clinical reasoning support middle-range theory development as well. What are some hypotheses you formed among relationships of activity intolerance, energy management, and effective ambulation? Didn't if–then thinking come in handy? Comparative analysis and reflexive comparison also come into play when considering where clients start and what progress they make. How did you use the thinking strategy of reflection check as you stopped to think?

MIDDLE-RANGE THEORY DEVELOPMENT CHALLENGE

Table 12-3 contains information about another set of diagnoses, interventions, and outcomes. This example relates to the diagnosis of nutrition—less than body requirements.

TABLE 12-3 Nutrition–Less Than Body Requirements; Building Links with OPT

DIAGNOSIS–NANDA	INTERVENTION–NIC	OUTCOME–NOC

Nutrition: Less than body requirements: inability to ingest or digest foods or absorb nutrients due to biological, psychological, or economic factors.
Indicators:
  Loss of weight with adequate food intake
  Body weight 20% or more under ideal
  Reported inadequate food intake
  Reported or evidence of lack of food
	1. Nutrition management: Assisting with or providing a balanced dietary intake of foods and fluids
	Activities:
	  Determine with dietitian the number of calories and type of nutrients needed
	  Adjust diet to client's lifestyle
	  Provide appropriate information
	2. Nutrition counseling: Use of an interactive helping process focusing on the need for diet modification
	Activities:
	  Eastablish a therapeutic relationship
	  Facilitate identification of eating behaviors to be changed
	  Establish short- and long-term goals for change
	  Discuss food buying habits
	3. Weight gain assistance: Facilitating gain of body weight
	Activities:
	  Discuss possible causes of low body weight
	  Monitor daily calories consumed
	  Assist with eating or feed client
	  Chart weight gain progress
		Nutritional status indicators
		Nutrient intake
		Biochemical measures (e.g., albumin)
		Body mass (e.g., body fat percent)
		Energy levels (e.g., stamina)
		Food and fluid intake (e.g., oral or tube feeding)
		Nutrient intake (e.g., caloric, protein)

Tables reprinted with permission from Blegen, M., & Tripp-Reimer, T. (1998). Implications of nursing taxonomies for middle-range theory development. *Advances in Nursing Science, 19*(3), 37–49.

Use the OPT model to think about relationships among the knowledge categories of diagnoses, interventions, and outcomes. Consider the frame to be middle-range theory development. Use the information in Table 12-3 and the structure of the OPT model to develop and think about a middle-range theory concerning interventions and outcomes around the diagnosis of nutrition—less than body requirements. What thinking strategies are you aware of using?

STOP AND THINK

1. **What are the outcome-present state-test conditions?**
2. **What elements require juxtaposing?**
3. **How will clinical decisions bridge the gap from present to desired state?**
4. **What evidence is needed to fill the gap?**
5. **When will clinical judgments be useful?**
6. **What kind of middle-range theory might you develop using this information as content and the OPT model as the structure?**
7. **Consider the survey list of prescriptive practice theory as you spin your middle-range theory.**

Use the Thinking Strategies Worksheet in Table 12-4 to note the thinking strategies you used as you reflected and reasoned about the elements of your middle-range theory. To what degree are these strategies part of your clinical reasoning repertoire?

SUMMARY

In this chapter the importance and need for practice to inform theory and research in nursing was discussed. Levels of practice theory were described. Building bridges among knowledge classification systems helps establish connections and propositions that create practice-relevant middle-range theories. The work that has been done over the past 10 years in knowledge classification system development has set the stage for middle-range theory development activities. Use of the OPT model and thinking strategies helps one develop, create, and reason about relationships and categories of knowledge that have practice relevance. Two examples about the development of middle-range theory were presented. Not every nurse needs to become a middle-range theorist. The raw ingredients for building and testing middle-range theories are made more explicit with the OPT model as a guiding structure.

TABLE 12-4 Thinking Strategies Worksheet for Middle-Range Theory Development

THINKING STRATEGY	DEFINITION	EXAMPLE FROM MIDDLE-RANGE THEORY CHALLENGE
Knowledge Work	Active use of reading, memorizing, drilling, writing, reviewing research, and practicing to learn clinical vocabulary	
Self-Talk	Expressing one's thoughts to one's self	
Schema Search	Accessing general and/or specific patterns of past experiences that might apply to the current situation	
Prototype Identification	Using a model case as a reference point for comparative analysis	
Hypothesizing	Determining an explanation that accounts for a set of facts that can be tested by further investigation	
If–Then Thinking	Linking ideas and consequences together in a logical sequence	
Comparative Analysis	Considering the strengths and weaknesses of competing alternatives	
Juxtaposing	Putting the present-state condition next to the outcome state in a side-by-side contrast	
Reflexive Comparison	Constantly comparing the client's state from time of observation to time of observation	
Reframing	Attributing a different meaning to the content or context of a situation based on tests, decisions, or judgments	
Reflection Check	Self-examination and self-correction of critical thinking skills and thinking strategies that support clinical reasoning	

KEY CONCEPTS

1. Nursing is a practice discipline that is supported by theory, research, and practice.

2. There are several levels of inquiry and practice theory that are useful for nursing. Factor isolating answers the question "What is this?" Factor relating asks, "What is happening here?" Situation relating theory poses the question "What will happen if . . . ?" Finally, situation producing or prescriptive theory helps answer the question, "How can I make . . . happen?"

3. Nursing prescriptions are enhanced by specification of a survey list that includes details regarding agency, client, framework, procedures, dynamics, and outcomes of prescriptions.

4. Nursing knowledge classification systems can be considered examples of factor isolating or level 1 practice theory. These systems answer the question "What is this?" and provide conceptual foundations for theory development and testing.

5. Building bridges among the knowledge classification systems requires critical, creative thinking and a structure for organizing the elements of knowledge classification systems.

6. The OPT model provides the structure for considering relationships among concepts across knowledge classification systems. The raw ingredients for building and testing middle-range theories are made more explicit with the OPT model as a guiding structure.

STUDY QUESTIONS AND ACTIVITIES

1. Retrieve one of the original articles on practice theory by Dickoff and James. Think about the ideas they present in light of what you know about nursing knowledge development activities in the past 30 years.

2. What middle-range concepts appeal to you in your current practice setting? Do you use a middle-range theory to guide your practice currently? Have you developed one based on experiences? How might you be able to formalize some of your ideas?

3. Conduct an internet search of literature in your area of interest. Include the term "middle-range theory" in your search. What do you discover? Share results of your search with peers and colleagues.

4. Pick a nursing diagnosis of interest to you. Create a table similar to the ones in this chapter. Include the diagnosis, interventions, and associated outcomes. Use the OPT model to structure these three classes of knowledge. Can you develop a middle-range theory from some of the concepts? How might you test your theory? What thinking strategies are most useful for this thinking exercise?

REFERENCES

Auvil-Novak, S. (1997). A middle-range theory of chronotherapeutic intervention for post surgical pain. *Nursing Research, 46*(2), 66–71.

Blegen, M., & Tripp-Reimer, T. (1997). Nursing theory, nursing research, and nursing practice: Connected or separate. In J. McClosky & H. Grace (Eds.), *Current issues in nursing* (5th ed., pp. 68–79. St. Louis, MO: Mosby.

Blegen, M., & Tripp-Reimer, T. (1998). Implications of nursing taxonomies for middle-range theory development. *Advances in Nursing Science, 19*(3), 37–49.

Chinn, P. (1994). *Developing substance: Mid-range theory in nursing.* Gaithersburg, MD: Aspen.

Dickoff, J., & James, P. (1968). A theory of theories: A position paper. *Nursing Research, 17*(3), 197–203.

Dickoff, J., James, P., & Widenback, E. (1968). Theory in a practice discipline. Part I: Practice oriented theory. *Nursing Research, 17*(5), 415–435.

Diers, D. (1979). *Research in nursing practice.* Philadelphia, PA: Lippincott.

Fawcett, J. (1995). *Analysis and evaluation of conceptual models of nursing* (3rd ed.). Philadelphia, PA: Davis.

Lenz, E. F., Pugh, L., Mulligan, R., Gift, A., & Suppe, F. (1997). The middle-range theory of unpleasant symptoms: An update. *Advances in Nursing Science, 19*(3), 14–27.

Morse, J. (1995). Exploring the theoretical basis of nursing using advanced techniques of concept analysis. *Advances in Nursing Science, 17*(3), 31–46.

Olson, J., & Hanchett, E. (1997). Nurse-expressed empathy, patient outcomes and development of a middle-range theory. *Image: The Journal of Nursing Scholarship, 29*(1), 71–76.

Polk, L. (1997). Toward a middle-range theory of resilience. *Advances in Nursing Science, 19*(3), 1–13.

Sternberg, R. (1985). Implicit theories of intelligence, creativity, and wisdom. *Journal of Personality and Social Psychology, 49,* 607–627.

Suppe, F. (1994). The nature of goal-directed theories and nursing practice theories. Paper presented at University of South Carolina College of Nursing, October.

Walker, L., & Avant, K. (1995). *Strategies for theory construction in nursing* (3rd ed.). Norwalk, CT: Appleton & Lange.

CHAPTER 13

Reasoning from the Past into the Future

COMPETENCIES

After completing this chapter, the reader should be able to:

1. Identify future health care industry trends.
2. Discuss the importance of clinical reasoning in identified health care trends.
3. Explain the need for a model of reasoning that is different than the nursing process.
4. Summarize the contributions of the OPT model to contemporary nursing practice.
5. Discuss the need for continued research and development of the OPT model and the clinical reasoning strategies presented in this text.

INTRODUCTION

In this chapter future trends and health care consequences are identified. Keeping up with future developments requires an investment in the development of clinical reasoning skills. The OPT model is a third-generation nursing process model that will make important contributions to future professional nursing practice. Use of the OPT model, Clinical Reasoning Web, and Thinking Strategies Worksheet defined and developed in this book will increase our understanding and development of more sophisticated clinical reasoning models. The advantages of the OPT model are summarized. The model is a useful structure for teaching clinical reasoning, and is also a guide for organizing the clinical supervision process. The model is a useful framework for organizing scholarship in terms of middle-range theory development and health services research. As more people learn and use the OPT model, research agendas are likely to develop. The art and science of clinical reasoning will continue to evolve.

FUTURE TRENDS AND HEALTH CARE CONSEQUENCES

Kaiser (1996), a health care futurist, notes we are a designer nation moving toward a designer health care system. Think for moment about the shifting trends we have witnessed as health care redesigns itself. There have been shifts from an obsession with disease to an interest and curiosity about health. There has been a shift from a focus on curing to healing. The industry is moving away from problem identification to outcome specification. Patient-centered systems replace provider-centered systems. Trends favor inclusion and networking rather than exclusion and isolation. There are shifts from competition to collaboration. People ask questions about ethics rather than profit. Community interest is a priority over self-interest. Community resources rather than institutional resources shape plans. Local responsibility is superseding federal responsibility. Innovation has replaced an emphasis on maintaining the status quo.

The scenarios that have been generated about the future of health are clear. Four major trends are evident: the globalization of health care; a focus on outcomes and cost-containment; an evolving information infrastructure; and the shift from a diagnose and treat to a predict and manage health care paradigm (Bezold & Mayer, 1996). This shift has tremendous consequences for nursing education, practice, and research. For example, what will nurses do when major chronic diseases can be identified in utero and then gene replacement therapy initiated so the disease no longer occurs? What are the consequences for nursing if people live to be 115 to 120 years old and are in good health? How will nursing interface with 24-hour health education and advances in telecognitive learning and telehealth and telemedicine?

One of the ways to stay abreast of these developments is to keep informed. Clinical reasoning is embedded in each of these trends. Maintaining and developing clinical reasoning skills is one way to master the changes inherent in future developments. The nursing profession brings compassion and understanding to the technological consequences of future health care predictions. Clinical reasoning requires one to

STOP AND THINK

1. **What thoughts and ideas do you have about the future of health care?**
2. **How well do you understand the consequences associated with the shift from diagnose and treat to predict and manage?**
3. **What is your current understanding of genetics, informatics, and telecommunications technology? Are you currently prepared to work and deal with the consequences of projected trends in genetics, informatics, telehealth, aging, and 24-hour telecommunication networks?**
4. **What role will clinical reasoning play in the projected health care future?**

think about the first-, second-, and third-order consequences of trends that are likely to influence patient care. Resourceful and resilient nurses need models of reasoning that build on the past and help them connect with the future.

Kaiser (1996) observes that we do not suffer from a resource problem in health care, but from design failure. Kaiser suggests a series of design parties where stakeholders come together to design a preferred future. Nurses must contribute to future health care design. Nurses need to attend design parties and bring professional optimism, curiosity, courage, and creativity to the table. Clinical reasoning will be a key ingredient in any design effort. Kaiser (1996) suggests the motto of the 21st century should be: "We are the problem, we are the solution, we are the resource." Clinical reasoning will remain important as health care providers tackle problems and create solutions.

THE OPT MODEL OF REFLECTIVE CLINICAL REASONING: CONTRIBUTIONS TO THE FUTURE OF HEALTH CARE

As the health care industry shifts to an outcomes orientation, the traditional nursing process needs modification. Knowledge workers of the future need new models of reasoning. A review of the history of nursing process points out significant changes over time (Pesut & Herman, 1998). The first generation of nursing process (1950–1970) focused on problems. The second generation (1970–1990) focused on diagnosis and reasoning. Each generation was influenced by the state of knowledge development and contemporary forces operative during its formation. The OPT model is a third-generation nursing process model that is a contribution to the future.

During the 1990s, tremendous progress was made in the area of nursing knowledge development. Nursing diagnoses, interventions, and outcomes provide the clinical vocabulary for clinical reasoning in nursing. Developments in nursing intervention classification systems and classification of nursing-sensitive patient outcomes require new models of reasoning. A different model can capitalize on nursing process heritage, accommodate recent knowledge development activities, and support contemporary practice. Furthermore, a new model of reasoning is likely to influence the development of middle-range theories in nursing and contribute to the creation of research-based practice.

At the heart of any new model is a practitioner's ability to engage in reflective critical thinking. It is impossible to think critically without thinking about your thinking. Metacognition is a key to critical thinking and clinical reasoning, as it contributes to an understanding of the thinking strategies involved in reflection. Metacognition or reflection is at the heart of the definition of critical thinking proposed by Facione and Facione (1996). Critical thinking is purposeful, self-regulatory judgment that gives reasoned consideration to evidence, context, conceptualizations, methods, and criteria (Facione & Facione, 1996).

The OPT model is a concurrent, iterative model of clinical reasoning that emphasizes reflective self-monitoring. This reasoning process results in framing a situation for the purpose of contrasting present-state data with outcome state criteria in order to make clinical decisions about nursing actions that bridge the gap so that clinical judgments can be made about outcome achievement. The OPT model "unpacks" some of the covert thinking processes nurses use as they reason. By making thinking strategies more explicit, it is possible to teach clinical reasoning more effectively.

The OPT model supports the third generation of nursing process (1990–2010) called outcome specification and testing (Pesut & Herman, 1998). The OPT model described in this book has several advantages over traditional nursing process models. First, the OPT model reinforces the reflective nature of clinical reasoning. Second, it captures the concurrent, iterative nature of clinical reasoning. Third, the model is more compatible with an outcome-focused health care system. Fourth, the model is built on a foundation of critical and creative thinking. Fifth, the model accommodates recent knowledge development activities in nursing. Finally, the model can be used in many settings for teaching, learning, conducting clinical supervision, theory development and testing, and organizing nursing research activities.

CLINICAL REASONING IN THE FUTURE: RESEARCH AND DEVELOPMENT

Based on our experiences we believe the OPT model is useful in clinical practice. As with any new development, people are more interested in evidence than experience. So there is a significant research and development challenge associated with the continued development of the OPT model. Several questions come to mind. To what degree does the model enhance client care and the achievement of outcomes? A research agenda in this area might include analysis and evaluation of client care outcomes comparing OPT and more traditional models. What cluster of clinical decisions (choice of interventions or nursing actions) lead to the optimal outcome in any condition? Are there instances when the OPT model would not be a useful way to organize thinking and reasoning? Using the OPT model as an organizing framework for evaluating relationships among data from the NMDS is a potential clinical research project. How can the OPT model articulate with current nursing information databases? What type of documentation system needs to be developed to accommodate use of the OPT model in clinical practice?

Additional research agendas can be developed in regard to middle-range theories. Middle-range theories that link knowledge from NANDA, NIC, and NOC can be designed and tested. Successful theories or best practices that result from such efforts can then serve as prototypes for future reasoning efforts and practice innovations. Defining a specific client or population condition and organizing nursing knowledge around the condition in terms of tests, clinical decisions, and clinical judgments is possible. Finally, do certain client states and clinical decisions require more or less reflection? How does the clinical supervision process contribute to the development of this increased reflective capacity? How is supervision using the OPT model different from traditional methods of supervision? Finally, what are the implications and consequences of using the OPT model for multi- and interdisciplinary care management and treatment planning?

If the OPT model was adopted, how might the education, teaching, and learning of students be different than it is today? How can faculty learn and use the OPT model? What are the curriculum revolution consequences of the OPT model? Educational research on reflection and the thinking strategies that support reflection is needed. How people learn to make choices (clinical decisions) and evaluate the meaning attributed to the results of a "test" needs investigation. The art of comparative analysis and reflexive comparison needs development.

Should nursing curricula teach NANDA, NIC, and NOC content as care knowledge? Should nursing curricula teach to prototypes? Attention to the knowledge work necessary to learn the facts associated with client conditions should be a prerequisite to clinical learning experiences. To what degree do textbooks need to be modified? Future texts might resemble compendiums of client stories with OPT analyses and solutions. Worksheets and workbooks that illustrate and assist students to see relationships among parts of the model with information from client stories would be useful teaching tools. Clinical Reasoning Webs and activities that help students identify keystone issues might accelerate learning and replace traditional nursing care plans. Routine use of the Thinking Strategies Worksheet would help students monitor their own thinking.

TOWARD A THEORY OF CLINICAL REASONING

There are many texts in nursing about critical thinking. In general these texts are valuable because they help students analyze and apply what we know today. The basic disadvantage of these texts is the fact that they are biased in favor of analytic intelligence at the expense of practical intelligence. Additionally, these texts do not help students master the systems thinking skills that are required for the future. As the profession gains knowledge, understanding, and experience, it will develop better theories about clinical reasoning. Such theories will help describe, explain, and predict elements of the reasoning process. Theories coupled with research will help us understand the science of clinical reasoning. Clinical practice, coupled with successful intelligence, will help us understand and appreciate the art of clinical reasoning. Experiment with the ideas presented in this book. Reflect, reason, and discover the art and science behind your own clinical reasoning.

SUMMARY

The health care industry is going through radical changes. Health care professionals must master and manage change. One way to master and manage change is to develop a systems thinking attitude and reflective clinical reasoning skills. Nursing has a long tradition of solving client care problems. However, a problem-solving model has limitations, especially in light of the outcome oriented care management demands of today.

As nursing science matures, the knowledge relevant to nursing practice expands. The OPT model of clinical reasoning is a structure that builds on nursing's heritage and uses knowledge gained to stimulate a systems way of thinking (Senge, 1990). Thinking does not happen by accident; it happens by intent. The activities and tools presented in this text were developed to provide new ways for nurses to intentionally reason about their practice.

The OPT model is an organizing conceptual framework. The notion of framing the client story is unique and makes explicit mental maps and models that nurses use on daily basis. The Clinical Reasoning Web is a new method and tool that supports reasoning about multiple client issues. The idea of a keystone issue is new. Identification of this issue during clinical reasoning episodes provides the nurse with an efficient and effective way to plan care. The thinking strategies that support the OPT model are proposed as the essential techniques of reflection. The fact that the model can use the knowledge contained in diverse classification systems demonstrates its potential as a universal template to structure reasoning.

Application of the model to several case studies across different contexts illustrated use of the model. The thinking strategies defined and applied systematically in each case, and across contexts, demonstrate the potential of the strategies to support clinical reasoning. The strategies are useful teaching and learning techniques.

Another example of the application of the model, tools, and strategies is in the area of clinical supervision. Relationships in the OPT model and questions used to guide thinking are fundamental to the reflection-in-action that is part of the learning involved in supervision experiences. Supervision contributes to the development of practical intelligence. Both academic and practical intelligence contribute to the development of nursing intelligence. The greater our nursing intelligence, the greater our understanding of the art and science of clinical reasoning.

KEY CONCEPTS

1. The health care industry is going through radical changes and will continue to change. Health care professionals must be prepared for this rapidly changing system. The one skill that will always be a central core of practice is the ability to engage in reflective clinical reasoning.

2. Thinking does not happen by accident, but by intent. The activities and tools presented in this text were developed to provide new ways for nurses to intentionally reason about their practice.

3. Clinical reasoning is necessarily embedded in many future health care predictions. The consequences of predicted trends have nursing education, practice, and research implications.

4. One of the ways to stay abreast of developments is to continue to practice clinical reasoning skills so that you will be prepared to master changes and consequences associated with reasoning about outcome specification, clinical decision making, and clinical judgments.

5. The OPT model is a third-generation nursing process model that is outcome-driven, builds on past generations of nursing process, and is concerned about outcome specification and testing.

6. Development of theories and design of research will help us understand the science and art of clinical reasoning.

7. Experiment with the ideas presented in this book so that you may discover and cherish the art and science behind your own clinical reasoning.

STUDY QUESTIONS AND ACTIVITIES

1. Is it important to have alternative reasoning models to the traditional nursing process? Why or why not?

2. Can you describe three ways the OPT model has influenced your clinical reasoning skills?

3. How, specifically, do you plan to use and evaluate the OPT model in your nursing practice?

4. How would the OPT model work in your place of employment or in agencies where you have had clinical learning experiences?

5. If you were to develop a documentation system to support the OPT model, what would it look like?

6. Can you identify other applications and uses for the OPT model? If so, write to us and let us know. We would be glad to collaborate with you on the development of your ideas.

REFERENCES

Bezold, C., Halperin, J., & Eng, J. (1993). *2020 visions: Health care information standards and technologies.* Rockville, MD: The United States Pharmacopeia Convention, Inc.

Bezold, C., & Mayer, E. (Eds.). (1996). *Future care responding to the demand for change.* New York: Faulkner & Gray.

Cetron, M. (1994). *An American Renaissance: 74 trends that will affect America's future and yours.* Bethesda, MD: World Future Society.

Facione, N., & Facione, P. (1996). Externalizing the critical thinking in knowledge development and clinical judgment. *Nursing Outlook, 44*(3), 129–136.

Kaiser, L. (1996). Designer healthcare for a designer nation: A new paradigm. In C. Bezold & E. Mayer (Eds.), *Future care responding to the demand for change* (pp. 189–218). New York: Faulkner & Gray.

Pesut, D., & Herman, J. (1998). OPT: Transformation of nursing process for contemporary practice. *Nursing Outlook, 46*(1), 29–36.

Senge, P. (1990). *The fifth discipline: The art and practice of the learning organization.* New York: Doubleday.

Sternberg, R. (1996). *Successful intelligence.* New York: Simon & Schuster.

Glossary

AACN—American Association of College of Nursing.

ANA—American Nurses Association.

Clinical Reasoning—reflective, concurrent, creative, and critical thinking processes embedded in practice used to frame, juxtapose, and test the match between a patient's present state and desired outcome state.

Clinical Reasoning Web—a pictorial representation of the functional relationships among diagnostic hypotheses derived from synthetic thinking that results in a convergence and identification of central issues that require care.

Clinical Vocabulary—knowledge classification systems that store nursing knowledge relevant to client care.

Comparative Analysis—process of considering the strengths and weaknesses of competing alternatives.

CPT—current procedural terminology.

Critical Thinking—purposeful self-regulatory judgment that results in interpretation, analysis, evaluation, and inference as well as the explanation of the evidential, conceptual, methodological, criteriological or contextual considerations upon which that judgment was based.

Critical Thinking Skills—skills of interpretation, analysis, inference, explanation, evaluation, and self-regulation.

Cue—sign, symptom, behavior, or characteristic displayed by a person that serves as data for clinical reasoning.

Cue Connection—the process of clustering two or more cues to form a pattern to guide framing, outcome specification, and establishment of a test.

Cue Logic—the deliberate structuring of client-in-context data to discern the meaning for client care. Can be deductive, inductive, or dialectic.

Decision Making—selecting interventions and actions that move clients from a presenting state to a specified or desired outcome state.

Deductive Reasoning—reasoning from general to specific.

DSM-IV—Diagnostic and Statistical Manual, 4th edition.

Framing—process of deriving the theme or meaning of a client-in-context situation. Framing results in mental models that influence and guide our perception and behavior.

Hypothesizing—determining an explanation that accounts for a set of facts and that can be tested by further investigation.

ICD—International Classification of Disease.

If–Then Thinking—linking ideas and consequences together in a logical sequence.

Inductive Reasoning—reasoning from specific to general.

Judgment—conclusions drawn from a test of the comparison of present state to a specified outcome state. Judgments result in conclusions, clinical decisions, reflection reframing or exit from a reasoning task.

Juxtaposing—side-by-side comparison of specified outcome-state criteria with present-state data.

Keystone Issue—central supporting element of the client's story that guides reasoning and care planning based on an analysis and synthesis of diagnostic possibilities as represented in a Clinical Reasoning Web.

Knowledge Work—active use of reading, memorizing, drilling, writing, reviewing research, and practicing to learn clinical vocabulary.

Metacognition—reflection.

NANDA—North American Nursing Diagnosis Association.

NIC—Nursing Interventions Classification (project).

NIQ—nursing intelligence quotient—the ability to apply what is learned from nursing care experiences and to use reasoning and inference effectively as a guide for the development of nursing care knowledge.

NOC—Nursing Outcomes Classification (project).

Outcome State—the desired condition of the client derived from the frame and initial present-state data as well as criteria that define the desired condition.

Outcome Specification—process of determining the desired end state of the client.

Outcome Focused Thinking—thinking that emphasizes outcomes or end results.

OPT (Outcome-Present State-Test) Model—A concurrent, iterative model of clinical reasoning that emphasizes reflective self-monitoring while framing the context and content of clinical reasoning and juxtaposing outcome state with present-state client data Clinical decision making in this model relates to choosing nursing actions Clinical judgment in this model is attributing meaning to the results of a test or match between desired criteriological outcome state and present state.

Present State—the initial condition of the patient derived from cue logic and defined by standardized taxonomic terms that change over time as a result of nursing actions and decisions as well as the current condition of the client at the time of the test.

Prototype Identification—using a model or textbook case as a reference point for comparative analysis.

Reflection—conscious application of the thinking strategies functional relationships of self-talk, prototype identification, schema search, hypothesizing, if–then thinking, juxtaposing, comparative analysis, reflexive comparison, and reframing.

Reflection Check—self-examination and self-correction of critical and creating thinking skills and thinking strategies that support clinical reasoning.

Reflection-in-action—the process by which professionals self-regulate thinking and action.

Reflexive Comparison—constantly comparing the client's state from time of observation to time of observation.

Reframing—attributing a different meaning to the content or context of a situation given a set of cues, tests, decisions, or judgments.

Retroduction—the process of reasoning using inductive data and deductive premises concurrently.

Schema—pattern imposed on complex reality or experience to assist in explaining it, mediating perception, or guiding a response.

Schema Search—accessing general and/or specific patterns of past experiences that might apply to the current situation.

Scenario—an outline of a hypothesized or projected chain of events.

Scenario Development—the process of developing a hypothesized or projected chain of events.

Self-Talk—expressing one's thoughts to one's self.

Spinning and Weaving a Web—the process of using thinking strategies to analyze and synthesize functional relationships among diagnostic hypotheses associated with a client's health status.

Test—the process of juxtaposing the present state and outcome state and evaluating the criteriological match between present state data and specified outcome; thinking strategies that support testing are comparative analysis and reflexive comparison.

Thinking Strategies—specific metacognitive techniques nurses use when engaged in reflective clinical reasoning.

OPT Model Worksheet

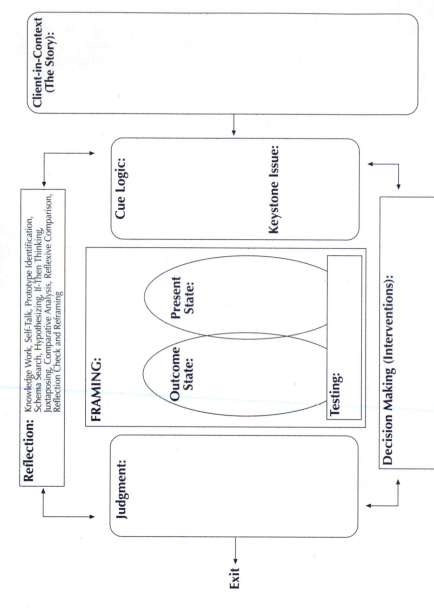

Client-in-Context (The Story):

Cue Logic:

Keystone Issue:

Reflection: Knowledge Work, Self-Talk, Prototype Identification, Schema Search, Hypothesizing, If-Then Thinking, Juxtaposing, Comparative Analysis, Reflexive Comparison, Reflection Check and Reframing

FRAMING:

Present State:

Outcome State:

Testing:

Decision Making (Interventions):

Judgment:

Exit

The OPT Model Worksheet

Index